Reforming Health Care

Reforming Health Care

The Philosophy and Practice of International Health Reform

Edited by

David Seedhouse

University of Auckland, New Zealand
and
University of Liverpool, UK

JOHN WILEY & SONS
Chichester · New York · Brisbane · Toronto · Singapore

Other Wiley Editorial Offices

John Wiley & Sons, Inc., 605 Third Avenue,
New York, NY 10158-0012, USA

Jacaranda Wiley Ltd, 33 Park Road, Milton,
Queensland 4064, Australia

John Wiley & Sons (Canada) Ltd, 22 Worcester Road,
Rexdale, Ontario M9W 1L1, Canada

John Wiley & Sons (SEA) Pte Ltd, 37 Jalan Pemimpin #05-04,
Block B, Union Industrial Building, Singapore 2057

Library of Congress Cataloging-in-Publication Data

Reforming health care: the philosophy and practice of international
    health reform/edited by David Seedhouse.
        p. cm.
    Most chapters reprinted with modifications from the journal Health
    care analysis.
        Includes bibliographical references and index.
        ISBN 0 471 95325 3
        1. Health care reform.   2. Health promotion.   I. Seedhouse,
    David.
        [DNLM: 1. Health Care Reform—trends—collected works.   2. Health
    Care Reform—standards—collected works.   3. Health Promotion—
    collected works.   4. National Health Progams—collected works.
    5. Cross-Cultural Comparison—collected works.   WA 540.1 R332   1995]
    RA394.R435   1995
    362.1—dc20
    DNLM/DLC
    for Library of Congress   94–44374
                                                                     CIP

British Library Cataloguing in Publication Data

A catalogue record for this book is available from the British Library

ISBN 0 471 95325 3

Typeset in 11/12 pt Plantin by Vision Typesetting, Manchester
Printed and bound in Great Britain by Redwood Books, Trowbridge, Wiltshire

Contents

List of Contributors   vii

Preface   ix

Introduction: The Logic of Health Reform   1
                 David Seedhouse

PART ONE: INTERNATIONAL HEALTH REFORM

Chapter 1.   Health Care Reform in the United States   15
              Chris Hackler

Chapter 2.   Oregon's Experiment   27
              Michael Brannigan

Chapter 3.   Health Care Reform in the United States: Clinton or
              Canada?
              Part One: The Clinton Reform Plan's Administrative
              Structure: The Reach and the Grasp   53
              Larry Brown and Theodore R. Marmor
              Part Two: Patterns of Fact and Fiction in the Use of
              Canadian Experience   60
              Theodore R. Marmor

Chapter 4.   Health Care Reform in the UK: Working for Patients?   71
              David Gladstone and Michael Goldsmith

Chapter 5.   From Evolution to Revolution: Restructuring the New
              Zealand Health System   85
              Toni Ashton

Chapter 6.   Choosing Core Health Services in The Netherlands   95
              Henk A.M.J. ten Have

Chapter 7.   Reforming Health Care in South Africa   101
              Michael Simpson

Chapter 8.   Health Care in Lithuania: From Idealism to Reality?   121
              Eugenijus Gefenas

PART TWO: BENEATH THE CRACKS—HEALTH REFORM AND SOCIAL JUSTICE

Chapter 9.   Going Off the Dole: A Prudential and Ethical Critique
of the 'Healthfare' State   131
Stuart F. Spicker

Chapter 10.   Health Reform and the Utopian Ideology of the New
Right   143
Michael Loughlin

Chapter 11.   Of Markets, Technology, Patients and Profits   149
Erich H. Loewy

Chapter 12.   Communitarian Illusions: Or Why the Dutch Proposal
for Setting Priorities in Health Care Must Fail   161
Theo van Willigenburg

Chapter 13.   Who should be Responsible for a Nation's Health?   167
Viola Schubert-Lehnhardt

Chapter 14.   A Turn for the Better? Philosophical Issues in
Evaluating Health Care Reforms   171
Alan Cribb

PART THREE: THE NEED FOR THEORY—A CASE STUDY IN THE PHILOSOPHY OF HEALTH PROMOTION

Chapter 15.   On the Nature and Ethics of Health Promotion. An
Attempt at a Systematic Analysis   185
Lennart Nordenfelt

Chapter 16.   The Borders of Health Promotion   199
Alan Cribb

Chapter 17.   Bad Faith and Victim-blaming: The Limits of Health
Promotion   209
Charles J. Dougherty

Chapter 18.   The Purpose–Process Gap in Health Promotion   221
Ian Buchanan

Conclusion   Theory before Practice?   229
David Seedhouse

Index   235

List of Contributors

Toni Ashton
Department of Community Health, School of Medicine, University of Auckland, Private Bag 91029, Auckland, New Zealand.

Michael C. Brannigan
Department of Philosophy, La Roche College, 9000 Babcock Boulevard, Pittsburgh, PA 15237, USA.

Lawrence D. Brown
School of Public Health, Columbia University, 600 West 168th Street, New York, NY 10032, USA.

Ian Buchanan
Health Promotion Adviser, Bury and Rochdale Health Authority, Staffing Offices, Birch Hill Hospital, Rochdale PL16 9QB, UK.

Alan Cribb
Centre for Educational Studies, King's College London, Cornwall House Annex, Waterloo Road, London SE1 8TX, UK.

Charles J. Dougherty
Center for Health Policy and Ethics, Creighton University, 2500 California Plaza, Omaha, Nebraska, USA.

Eugenijus Gefenas
Institute of Philosophy, Sociology and Law, Tuskulenu 13–1, 2051 Vilnius, Lithuania.

David Gladstone
Department of Social Policy, University of Bristol, 8 Woodland Road, Bristol BS8 1TN, UK.

Michael Goldsmith
Sedgwick Noble Lowndes Health Care Ltd., Sedgwick House, The Sedgwick Centre, London E1 8DX, UK.

Chris Hackler
University of Arkansas for Medical Sciences, College of Medicine, Division of Medical Humanities, 4301 West Markham, Mail Slot 646, Little Rock, Arkansas, USA.

Erich H. Loewy
The University of Illinois College of Medicine at Peoria, Department of Medicine, Box 1649, Peoria, Illinois 61658–1649, USA.

Michael Loughlin
Manchester Metropolitan University, Crewe and Alsager College, Hassall Road, Alsager, Cheshire ST7 2HL, UK.

Theodore Marmor
Yale University, School of Organisation and Management, 135 Prospect Street, Box 1A, Yale Station, New Haven, Connecticut 06520, USA.

Lennart Nordenfelt
Department of Health and Society, University of Linköping, S–581 83 Linköping, Sweden.

Viola Schubert-Lehnhardt
Martin-Luther Universitat Halle Wittenberg, Bereich Medizin, Abteilung Ethik und Geschichte der Medizin, Postfach 0–4010 Halle, Germany.

Michael A. Simpson
Department of Psychiatry, Medical University of Southern Africa, PO MEDUNSA 0204, South Africa.

Stuart F. Spicker
Visiting Professor, Center for Ethics, Medicine and Public Issues, Baylor College of Medicine, Houston, Texas 77030, and Professor Emeritus, University of Connecticut School of Medicine, USA.

Henk A.M.J. ten Have
Department of Ethics, Philosophy and History of Medicine, Catholic University of Nijmegen, PO Box 9101, 6500 HB Nijmegen, The Netherlands.

Theo van Willigenburg
Center for Bioethics and Health Care, Faculty of Theology, Heidelberglaar 2, 3584 CS Utrecht, The Netherlands.

Preface

Health reform has been the subject of widespread social concern throughout the present decade. At the time of writing there is little sign that this trend will diminish. Indeed, in some countries health reform receives so much attention that it has become an ever-present feature of public debate. But all trends have their day, however permanent they may seem, and any genuine reform process must come to an end. How will the 1990s health reforms turn out? Will the reformers be satisfied with their work? Will the public enjoy highly cost-effective health systems offering the best available health benefits? Or are the health reforms bound to fail?

To study health reform it is essential to know what is actually happening to and within various health systems. But to be aware of the facts alone is not enough. Philosophical questions must be addressed if health reform is to be explored in any depth. What, for instance, *is* a health reform? What is a health system? What are—and what ought to be—the typical goals of the health reform process? And by what criteria is the success or failure of health reform to be assessed?

This collection of articles is intended to enhance the understanding of health reform, and to play a modest part in resolving the current international obsession with the subject. *Reforming Health Care* is by no means comprehensive (either in its international scope, or in its description of the minutiae of health policy) but it does offer an informed view of the 'health debates' currently taking place in eight countries. The book includes two articles which comprehensively describe the reasons why health reform is thought to be so urgently required in the US (and why Canadians are far less anxious to reform their system); an illuminating and detailed account of the oft-cited, but far less often understood, 'Oregon Experiment'; an admirably uncomplicated description of recent changes in the British National Health Service; an explanation of the radical reforms made to the New Zealand health system; two Dutch views of health reform; a disturbing description of the legacy of apartheid now facing South African health reformers; and two contributions which offer an insight into the emerging 'post-socialist' perception of health services.

In addition the book offers the reader a grasp of the theoretical fundamentals of health reform. Parts Two and Three add philosophical substance to the policy discussion which forms the bulk of Part One. Part Two, as its title suggests, makes it clear that any proposal to reform a 'health system' must stand upon some conception of social justice. And Part Three illustrates, by means of a 'case study' from the philosophy of health promotion, that a theory of health reform is indispensable if health care is to be systematically improved.

Moreover, in the editorial sections, an attempt is made to indicate the essential nature of health reform, and to show how it is only by understanding its logical structure that burgeoning 'health reform initiatives' can be properly managed.

It should be noted that most of the book's chapters have already appeared in *Health Care Analysis: Journal of Health Philosophy and Policy*. The majority of them have been modified, at least slightly, in order to be included, and one is the unedited original of a paper which appeared in the first issue of the journal. It was felt that these writings are of such interest that, with the addition of fresh editorial analysis and the inclusion of some specially commissioned material, the collection merited publication as a book for the widest possible distribution.

David Seedhouse
University of Auckland
New Zealand

Introduction: The logic of Health Reform

Philosophy and Practice

Although philosophy has much to contribute to health reform its advantages are rarely appreciated by health care policy-makers. To most pragmatists the philosopher who tries to suggest a way forward in social reality is like an aerial cartographer crash-landed in a jungle—his skills irrelevant in an alien context. It can seem that philosophy has nothing to offer to help solve immediate problems, and so it is frequently ignored altogether.

So great is the gap between the purity of philosophical reasoning and the messy manoeuvring required to change human organisations that it can seem that philosophy and down-to-earth policy-making are simply worlds apart. A political philosopher may offer the most lucid egalitarian theory;[1] a health economist may give an exacting account of a system designed to allocate scarce health care resources to maximum effect;[2] yet the fact is that such ideas—however strenuously they are thought through and however clearly they are put—can never work in the world as it really is. If elegant philosophical theories are to succeed the world as a whole has to run along equally elegant lines. And of course it does not.

But although this pessimistic view of applied philosophy is not easy to refute, it is equally hard to see how philosophical analysis can be entirely disregarded by planners who wish to avoid inconsistent policy-making. Unless a reformer has first thought out what she means by reform, and defined those principles she considers should guide the practical reform process, she cannot even begin to make cogent changes. Study of what passes for health reform in some countries makes it clear that many 'reformers' have undertaken only the barest minimum of philosophical reflection, if they have done any at all.[3,4] Transformations are undoubtedly taking place within and to health services, but they are almost always based on incomplete thinking, and are often being made for 'sets' of reasons which do not make sense. In those places[5,6] where there has been more contemplation about the ends of health reform, the reforms tend to have stronger justifications. But even the best examples have not been thought through with philosophical rigour.

In some of the chapters of this book philosophy and practice really do seem worlds apart. As Michael Simpson points out the facts and figures of apartheid, as Michael Brannigan describes the lengthy legislation which preceded the 'Oregon Experiment', and as Theodore Marmor reflects on the political and practical pros and cons of the many US proposals for health reform, philosophical considerations can seem far away. But though they are not always prominent they are nevertheless always there: arguments against apartheid must rest on an alternative theory of social justice, the 'Oregon Experiment' makes the fundamental assertion that human beings are of equal value, and the US health reform debate becomes properly focused only when it is seen as a product of conflicting social philosophies.

In what follows an attempt is made to demonstrate something of the logic of this philosophical base, and to show that philosophical analysis is essential to cogent health reform. This is not to say that philosophy has all the answers. But it is to argue that an understanding of the logical structure of health reform is a prerequisite for rational planning, and that philosophy is uniquely placed to describe it. Unless this logical structure is understood health reform must be a hit and miss affair, and the would-be health reformer will be left in roughly the same position as a motor mechanic who does not understand the overall structure and purpose of a car engine. The mechanic will be able to tinker here and there, but without a general theoretical grasp of what she is doing will most likely do more harm than good.

The Nature of Reform

To comprehend the logic and nature of 'health reform' it is first necessary to distinguish the general characteristics of *any* reform process.

What is a Reform?

In general, *any reform must aim to reconstruct an existing structure or system in order to enable it to achieve its original end(s) in an improved way.* A clothes manufacturer who reforms his factory may decide to buy new machinery, or to employ his staff differently, or to use more durable material—but he must still aim to produce clothes. This is a simple point, but it is nevertheless of fundamental importance to the understanding of health reform.

Five conditions for practical reform are implied by the above definition. These are:

1. The area of activity which is to be reformed must be delineated.
2. The originally desired overall purposes of the delineated activities must be known (even if the activities are not presently achieving the desired purposes).
3. It must be clear why the existing set-up is:
   a. not achieving the desired overall purpose(s) or
   b. is achieving the desired overall purpose(s) but with the disadvantage(s) X, Y, Z . . . (which must themselves be clearly defined).
4. Strategies to deal with (3a) or (3b) must be both known and possible. It must be clear how the intended reforms will ensure that the desired overall purposes will be better achieved.

5. The originally desired overall purposes should not be abandoned (though, dependent on delineation, the purposes of some sub-systems might be changed). To do this would not be to reform but to implement radical change (which is what the clothes manufacturer would do if he closed down his factory and used the premises to open up a natural history museum instead).

These conditions are essential for the systematic reform of any system, and can be translated into a set of questions to the reformer:

1. What is the area of activity that is to be reformed?
2. What are the original desired overall purposes of the delineated activities?
3. Why is the existing set-up:
   a. not achieving these desired purposes, or
   b. achieving the purposes at the unwanted and unnecessary cost of X, Y, Z?
4. How is/are (3a) and/or (3b) to be addressed?

Reforming a Commercial System

In the case of a commercial system it is very easy to see how the above questions might be answered. For example, consider very briefly the case of reform of a car manufacturing enterprise. Any of the many 'sub-systems', or the 'grand business system' as a whole, may be open to reform. Whatever the case, the desired overall purpose(s) of any delineated systems must be stated (and, of course, the purpose(s) of the grand business system must always be made clear since these must influence those of the sub-systems). If, for instance, the ultimate purpose of the grand system is said to be to 'maximise financial profit', and if two of the purposes of a particular sub-system under inspection are 'maintaining safety standards' and 'devising ways to attract customers', then it might be decided to build vehicles using metals that are lighter, but equally strong, and which cost the same, as the metals used in the existing production process: lighter metals would increase the maximum speed of the cars, decrease petrol consumption, be as safe as the metals used previously, and—in theory—attract more customers.

Of course, like all complex grand systems, the purposes of business systems are not necessarily compatible. Sometimes, and under some delineations, they will be consistent, but at other times they will conflict. A manager of a business, for example, may have a genuine desire to offer the longest possible guarantees on electrical appliances, and to offer maximum assistance to customers having difficulty understanding their instruction manuals—even to the point of employing 'special installation assistants'. And this combination of purposes may work very well in some circumstances. However, perhaps under pressure of economic recession, the manager's helpful policy may turn out to be too expensive, in which case it would inevitably be modified by the overriding business purpose—to maximise financial profit.

In practice, the reform of a business must involve the restructuring of many

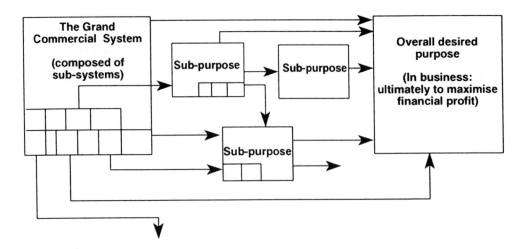

Figure 1   The basic components of a commercial system as a reformer might see them (Boxes and arrows illustrative only)

more inter-reacting sub-systems, and the calculations of reformers of commercial systems can become highly complex. However, although Figure 1 is undoubtedly a massive oversimplification, it does illustrate the basic contours of commercial reform.

The logic of 'business reform' is plain to see. If 'maximising profit' is the goal of the system, then a comprehensive reform will reassess every part of that system in order to discover if any part of it can be restructured so as to make more—or lose less—money. However, where the system under scrutiny is not indisputably a business, its reform becomes a considerably greater challenge.

A Brief Discussion of a Reform Process in a not Wholly Commercial System: Reform of a National Railway System

Consider a national railway system, and how it might be reformed. The grand system might be defined as:

> the physical existence and function of all trains, rolling stock, tracks, stations, staff and other assets under the direct financial/legal control of the system's directors

(the 'directors' may or may not be defined as part of the system) and its 'overall desired purposes' said to be:

1. To offer a convenient service to passengers.
2. To attract as many customers as possible.
3. To make as much financial profit as possible.
4. Not to damage the environment.

(In reality there may well be several further general purposes).

Given these clarifications the area(s) to be reformed might be variously delineated. For example, the scope of the reforms might be defined as: the entire system; the passenger service; the goods service; safety; the pricing of tickets, some combination of these, or many other possibilities.

Unlike a wholly commercial system, a national railway system with the above four ends does not have a single dominant purpose. And this fact makes any attempt at reform hugely complicated. On the face of it it may seem that the cheaper the ticket prices, and the more accessible the railway stations, the more passengers there will be. However, while cheaper fares and more stations may be highly convenient for passengers (purpose 1 above), such a policy may neither maximise profits (purpose 3) nor protect the environment (purpose 4). It might, for instance, be the case that certain services (perhaps early morning trains to big cities) are in great demand from wealthy passengers, who can afford and are willing to pay premium prices. And it might also be the case that to keep prices low train maintenance has to be reduced, so causing increased air and noise pollution. In such circumstances purposes (1) and (3), and (3) and (4) (at least) will be in conflict. In a system with multiple overall purposes reform of one delineated general purposive area can have a negative effect on another delineated general purposive area. In such systems, if reforms are not based on a hierarchy of reasoned principles, then:

1. The reason for and justification of the reforms will be *fudged*. The aim overall will be said to be to 'improve things all round', but if the question of the 'overall desired purpose' of a complex system is fudged then sooner or later incompatible proposals for reform will be put forward (though this may not always be easy to see) and actual reforms will conflict.

Or,

2. One of the desired purposes may become *unduly predominant*. For instance, in the case of reform of a railway system 'maximising profit' might come to take absolute precedence over comfort and safety (or vice versa—though this seems unlikely these days). If so, then as this purpose grows in significance and control, so the other purposes will diminish in importance.

Or,

3. An *inappropriate* purpose may become predominant. That is, a purpose which the system was never meant to have (or conceptually cannot have) may either be 'smuggled in' or be an unintended consequence of a muddled reform process. For instance, if the railway system 'reformers' were to decide to cut railway services, to sell assets, and to move into the hotel and leisure industry, this would not be a reform. If it were said to be one this would be both a conceptual and practical error.

It might be argued, against this point, that the definition of reform offered earlier (see p. 2) is too restrictive. It might be claimed that 'reform' not only means restructuring, but can mean the radical rethinking of goals as well. But this stretches the definition of 'reform' too far. For instance, if it were to be suggested that, as part of a prison reform, prisons should have the sole purpose of 'rehabilitation' (and should therefore no longer punish prisoners) then this would be to suggest something substantially more than reform. It would be to suggest a quite different *raison d'être* for prisons, and would alter the very meaning of the term 'prisoner' (potential 'prisoners' would have to *volunteer* for prison rehabilitation!).

And even if such an extreme view of reform were to be allowed, any 'reform' would still have to refer ultimately to a well-developed account of 'overall desired purpose'. If 'reform' can in fact mean 'changing some or all of the purposes of a system', then this serves only to import an additional requirement to say why the original purposes were wrong or inadequate in the first place.

As any business person and first year economist knows, in order to reform any system sensibly its various purposes must be ranked in order of priority, they must be balanced consistently against each other, clear plans must be formed and tested, and it must, at some point, be demonstrated that the restructuring of the system leads to the enhanced achievement of the original ends. All this is strikingly obvious, and entirely possible in a commercial enterprise. However, in state-owned railway systems—or in systems which are partly for profit and partly for service—it is a different story. Exactly the same logic applies, but reformers face intractable practical problems for the simple reason that the overall purpose of the system is either not clear, or is disputed.

In the case of reform of a railway system the basic contours of reform look like those shown in Figure 2.

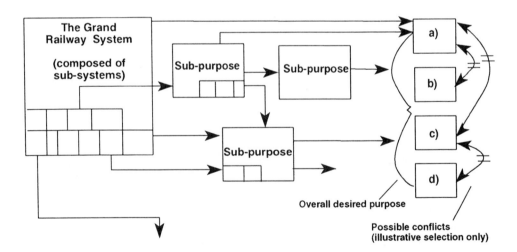

Figure 2   The basic components of a national railway system as a reformer might see them.   Purposes (a)–(d) are all said to be vital purposes of a railway system. The tendency is either for their relative status to be fudged, for one to become unduly dominant, or for an inappropriate 'governing purpose' to be imported.

First: It is assumed that

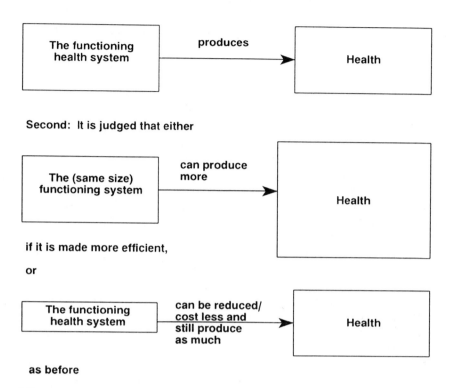

Second: It is judged that either

if it is made more efficient,

or

as before

Figure 3   A common view of health reform

Reforming a Health Service

Figure 3 shows a very simple characterisation of the contemporary view of health reform.

This characterisation only makes practical sense if:

1. The 'functioning health system' is delineated and understood in reality.
2. 'Health' (the supposed 'output' of the 'health system') is both defined and can be assessed.

(This is simply a different way of saying that the characterisation makes sense only if 'the five conditions for practical reform' are actually met (see pp. 2–3).)

But in fact neither (1) nor (2) is the case. Both (1) and (2) can be explained in different ways, and this means that the process and outcome of 'health reform' will be different (perhaps hugely different) dependent on how these two aspects are described.[7] The trouble (for the would-be health reformer) is that the definition of 'overall desired purpose' (or 'health') and the delineation of the 'health system' are dependent variables. Some thinkers define 'health' very broadly,[8,9] others define 'health' much more narrowly.[10,11] For some 'health' is possible only if a person can achieve her 'vital goals'[9] while for others a person is healthy so long as she is 'clinically normal',[10] regardless of whether she finds her life satisfying or not. Equally, there are numerous ways to understand a 'health system'. For some a health system can be entirely explained by reference to hospital services and their satellite medical systems; for some a health system includes not only medical endeavours but also activities such as community care and health promotion; while for others a health system incorporates all systems designed to enable people to live healthy lives. At one end of the spectrum health systems are thought to be simply the set of medical processes—at the other end, since so much of the social world has an impact on people's health (however it is defined), health systems are considered to be synonymous with general welfare provision.

If a 'health system' had only one 'overall desired purpose' then reform might be a relatively straightforward matter. In such circumstances, the task of health reform might be analogous to the task of reforming a commercial business. If, for instance, the 'health system' had the sole overall purpose of eradicating disease, and could have an entirely free hand to do this, then the task would merely be to work out ways to eradicate ever more diseases (and the results of these calculations would, of themselves, act to delineate the system). But no health system has the luxury of such single-mindedness—in the real world even a health system thought of as a 'disease eradication service' would have to take account of financial costs and the interests of competent citizens, at the very least—and this would, at a stroke, complicate matters enormously. To eradicate some diseases (lung cancer and ischaemic heart disease for instance) might conceivably cost more than a nation's gross national product. In practice, a balance between disease eradication and reasonable budgeting would clearly have to be drawn. Equally clearly, the interests of some citizens might conflict with the purpose of the single-minded system, so requiring further compromise (see Figure 4).

The great conceptual (and so practical) problem presently facing would-be health reformers is that even if the health system is defined in the narrowest sense, as (state controlled) 'hospital services and their satellite medical systems', then it automatically has very many purposes—and no obviously predominant one. And it is simply not clear which of these purposes are merely 'sub-system purposes' and which are 'overall desired purposes'. To make matters yet worse, just as with the railway system these purposes do not always gel together, and can often conflict. For example, see Figure 5.

In certain contexts conflicts can occur between (b) and (c) (a standard problem of traditional medical ethics), (a) and (j) (the patient may define 'effective' in an alternative way—preferring conservation of a limb rather than the surgical removal of a tumour, for instance), (a) and (d) (not everyone can always obtain (a) in a 'cash-limited' system), (a) and (e), (e) and (f), (d) and (f), (c) and (g), and so on. What is more, if it is stated that a purpose of the health system is 'to minimise financial cost' (a consideration not listed in Figure 5), then many of the tensions are instantly heightened.

The US health reform debate illustrates this conundrum in reality. The

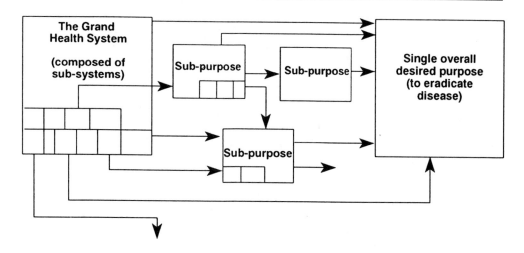

Figure 4   This is not and cannot be the case

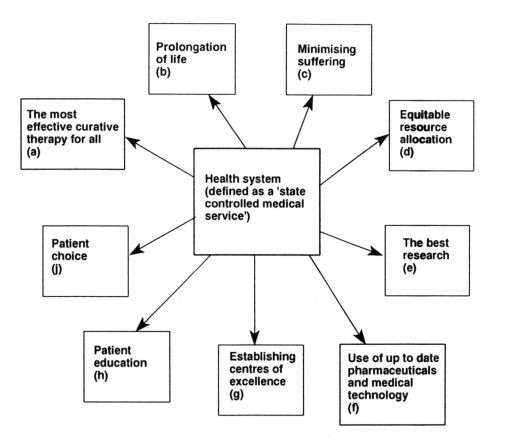

Figure 5   Possible purposes of a narrowly defined health system

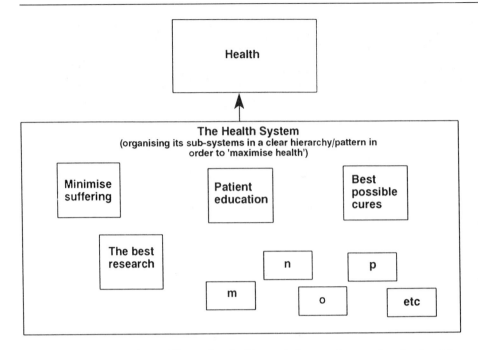

Figure 6   'Health' used hypothetically to define and organise the health system

Clinton reforms are supposed to bring about better health (although health is never properly defined), lower costs, ensure universal access, guarantee comprehensive treatment, and enable rational resouce distribution and the definition of a just set of 'core health services'. But, assuming accepted US definitions of these terms, logic shows that not all these goals can be achieved simultaneously, and particularly not if cost-control is the predominant factor.

It is, of course, theoretically possible to solve this problem by ranking purposes in order of importance (and therefore changing the delineation of 'the system'). However, to do this it is necessary to have a 'super-purpose' which can organise and define the hierarchy. And the only likely nominal candidate for such a role is 'health', see Figure 6. But this is going in circles. 'Health' needs to be defined in order to perform its 'governing' or organising role—yet it is defined only by very few 'health reformers', and then never with philosophical depth.

A theory of health is obviously required for rational, theory-based health reform. In the absence of a philosophical theory of health to govern health reform the existing 'health system' 'rushes in' to fill the theoretical vacuum, and health is defined by philosophical default. And in fact it is at the moment widely believed that the prevailing 'health system' and its workings adequately define 'health'. But, because the 'health system' is almost always taken to be a 'medical system' (and usually a medical system dominated by hospital services) by contemporary health reformers, and because the 'medical system' is always the product of historical accident and political compromise, the 'theory of health' it creates is correspondingly inconsistent and incoherent—and so not really a theory at all. Health reform turns out either to be reform dominated by the single purpose of reducing fiscal cost, or reform inspired only by theories of purpose generated by the supposedly ailing system itself. And if this analysis is correct then—for all the ingenuity and good intentions of some health reformers—the prospects for 1990s health reform are bleak.

In none of the projects described in this book are the five conditions for practical reform fully met, and sometimes they are not met at all. Perhaps this is unavoidable. Perhaps the conditions are nothing more than the demands of an academic philosopher who does not have to make the hard choices. However—whether or not the five conditions ask too much of workers on the ground—if the conditions are not met then the citizens of those countries at present experimenting with 'health reform' are entitled to ask what is going on, because—to the extent that the conditions are not met—it is not reform. Moreover, if it turns out that the political reality of health planning means that the five conditions can never realistically be met, then perhaps the entire project should be re-assessed. The chapters which follow may help prompt a decision.

References

1. Norman, R. (1987). *Free and Equal: A Philosophical Examination of Political Values*, Oxford University Press, Oxford.
2. Culyer, A. (1992). The morality of efficiency in health care—some uncomfortable implications. *Health Economics*, 1(1), 7–18.
3. Gladstone, D. and Goldsmith, M. (1994). Health care reform in the UK: working for patients. In, *Reforming Health Care: The Philosophy and Practice of International Health Reform*, ed. by D. Seedhouse, John Wiley & Sons, Chichester.
4. Simpson, M. (1994). Reforming health care in South Africa. In, *Reforming Health Care: The Philosophy and Practice of International Health Reform*, ed. by D. Seedhouse, John Wiley & Sons, Chichester.
5. ten Have, A.M.J. (1994). Choosing core health services in the Netherlands. In, *Reforming Health Care: The Philosophy and Practice of International Health Reform*, ed. by D. Seedhouse, John Wiley & Sons, Chichester.
6. Brannigan, M. (1994). Oregon's experiment. In, *Reforming Health Care: The Philosophy and Practice of International Health Reform*, ed. by D. Seedhouse, John Wiley & Sons, Chichester.
7. Cribb, A. (1994). A turn for the better? Philosophical issues in evaluating health care reforms. In, *Reforming Health Care: The Philosophy and Practice of International Health Reform*, ed. by D. Seedhouse, John Wiley & Sons, Chichester.
8. Seedhouse, D.F. (1986). *Health: The Foundations for Achievement*, John Wiley & Sons, Chichester.
9. Nordenfelt, L. (1987). *On the Nature of Health*, D. Reidel, Dordrecht.
10. Boorse, C. (1981). On the distinction between disease and illness. In, *Concepts of Health and Disease: Interdisciplinary Perspectives*, ed. by A.L. Caplan, H.T. Englehardt Jr. and J.J. McCartney, Addison-Wesley, Massachusetts.
11. Veatch, R.M. (1981). The medical model: its nature and problems. In, *Concepts of Health and Disease: Interdisciplinary Perspectives*, ed. by A.L. Caplan, H.T. Englehardt Jr. and J.J. McCartney, Addison-Wesley, Massachusetts.

Part One:
International Health Reform

Chapter 1

Health Care Reform in the United States

Chris Hackler

University of Arkansas for Medical Sciences, Division of Medical Humanities,
Little Rock, Arkansas, USA

The Problem

Rising Costs

Health care expenditure has increased over the past two decades by an average
of 11.6% per year, considerably higher than the overall rate of inflation of
8.7%.[1] Health care spending in the US for 1992 was US$838.5 billion, over
14% of the gross domestic product (GDP). The previous director of the Office
of Management and Budget testified before Congress that without serious
structural changes, health care would account for 17% of the GDP by 2000 and
37% by 2030.[2] These estimates now appear conservative. Older Americans
spent 10.6% of their after-tax income on health care in 1961, before the
enactment of Medicare (which provides most of the cost of health care for all
citizens over the age of 65). In 1991, even with the help of Medicare, their
out-of-pocket expenses consumed 17.1% of their income.[3]

Individual consumers are not the only ones affected by escalating health care
costs. Increased government outlays through Medicare and Medicaid (the
federal health care assistance programme for the poor) exacerbate the federal
deficit. To control expenditures the government has reduced Medicare benefits,
paid only a portion of Medicaid bills, and imposed a prospective payment
scheme based on averages rather than actual costs. The real cost of providing
care has not diminished in proportion to the lower levels of reimbursements
now paid to physicians and hospitals. Consequently the surplus costs have been
shifted from public to private payers. Such cost shifting has further accelerated
the increasing cost of health insurance for individuals and the cost of health

Reforming Health Care: The Philosophy and Practice of International Health Reform.
Edited by D. Seedhouse. © 1995 John Wiley & Sons Ltd.

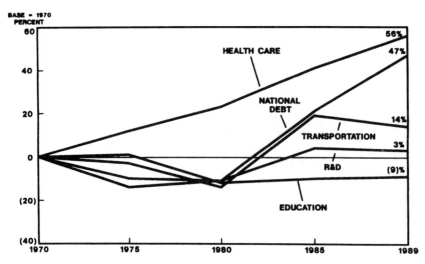

Figure 1   Trend of health care costs and other sector expenditures as a percentage of GNP. (From the *Journal of Medicine and Philosophy*, with permission.[5])

coverage for businesses, putting them at a competitive disadvantage. Chrysler Corporation estimates that health care costs, including those of its suppliers, added US$700 to the cost of each vehicle in 1989, about three times the added cost in Japan ($246) and Canada ($223). Ford Motor Company spends much more on health care than it does on steel.[4] As more of our money goes to health care, less is available for other critical social needs, such as education and economic investment (Figure 1 shows the change in outlay for some of these items).[5]

There are many reasons for this relentless rise in the cost of health care. Malpractice insurance premiums continue to climb, reflecting increasing litigation and higher awards. Patient education and preventive medicine receive little reward under the current system, which focuses on curing rather than avoiding illness. The cost of care is not addressed in medical education, so that physicians rarely know the cost of a test or procedure they order. This fact reflects a more pervasive attitude. As consumers we expect and demand the highest level of care available, which we equate with the most intensive, extensive or expensive. We tend to think of medical care as an absolute priority, not subject to the cost–benefit comparisons that usually structure our economic choices. Moreover, since our bills are usually paid by third parties, there is little incentive for either consumers or providers to control spending. As a result, our hospitals spend vast amounts building, remodelling and purchasing the latest technology in competition for patients. For example, there are 10 000 mammogram machines in the US, while only 2000 would be necessary to meet current demand, and 5000 would screen the entire population.[6] Without a doubt a more rational deployment of resources would significantly reduce total health care outlay.

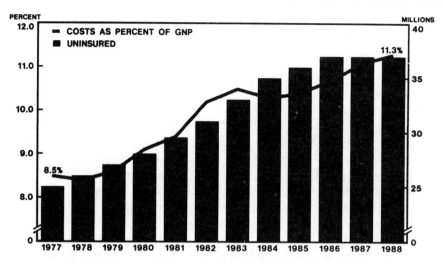

Figure 2   Health care costs and the uninsured 1977–1988, USA. — Costs as percent of GNP; ■ uninsured. (From the *Journal of Medicine and Philosophy*, with permission.[5])

Limited Access

Americans who can afford it receive the technologically most advanced medical care in the world. Our formidable challenge is to preserve the quality of available care while gaining control over runaway costs and at the same time including all of our citizens in the system. It is clear that the problems of cost and access are related. Most obviously, fewer are able to afford insurance as the cost rises (Figure 2 illustrates this correlation).[7] A recent study by the Agency for Health Care Policy and Research of the Department of Health and Human Services has found that 20% of the population of the US had no health insurance for some or all of 1987. Over 24 million were uninsured for the entire year, and another 23 million for part of the year. An estimated 50 million more are underinsured, with policies that provide inadequate coverage (a major illness could produce bankruptcy). Medicaid, the public assistance programme for indigent patients, covers only the poorest of the poor in most states. The majority of these without coverage are the working poor and their dependents. Many small businesses cannot afford to offer health insurance, and several larger and more prosperous companies avoid the expense by hiring mostly part-time workers. Self-employed, seasonal, and temporary workers may also lack coverage.

The uninsured often receive inadequate care under humiliating conditions. Many physicians refuse to take uninsured patients, and some even refuse to take patients with Medicaid coverage. Individuals may not be able to obtain important elective procedures until their needs become acute. At this point they may go to expensive emergency rooms where they cannot be turned away. If they are unable to pay for their care, the cost is shifted to insured patients, further increasing the cost of premiums—another example of the inextricable link between cost and access.

Proposed Solutions

Incremental Revision

A conservative approach to reform might attempt to control costs and increase access by modifying the present patchwork system and encouraging individuals to be more circumspect and parsimonious in their consumption of health care services. To expand access, underwriting practices could be regulated so that fewer individuals are denied coverage or thrown into prohibitively expensive risk pools. Medicaid could be extended to cover the 'uninsurable' (those who are already in poor health). Managed care options in the private sector, such as health maintenance organisations or preferred provider arrangements, could be promoted in an effort to control costs. Individuals could be encouraged to accept more modest levels of care rather than demanding the best and most expensive care available. Advance directives could be promoted as a way of controlling wasteful end-of-life expenditures. In addition to the usual language that refuses life-prolonging treatment, clauses could be added to directives authorising physicians and family to consider the cost of treatment, and might explicitly reject expensive procedures that do not have corresponding benefits. Discounts might even be offered by insurance companies as an incentive to complete an advance directive.

However, it is highly doubtful that sufficient savings could be realised from managed care and voluntary restraint to offset the added cost of extending access. Managed care has not had great success thus far in containing health care costs. Increased use of advance directives is unlikely to help significantly; patients who receive sustained intensive care before death account for only about 1% of total annual Medicare cost. Volume appears to be much more important in determining overall health care costs. Rather than so-called 'heroic medicine' it is the repetition of comparatively 'small ticket' items, and the needs of the chronically ill that are largely responsible for rising expenditures.[8] In general, it seems naive to expect most Americans to request or voluntarily to accept a lower level of care than their coverage allows. Indeed, it seems unfair to reduce costs by encouraging sacrifice from the altruistic while others continue a more extravagant consumption of resources.

In the long run we must moderate our strong individualist orientation and embrace a more communitarian ethic, but reform of the health care system cannot wait for such a conversion. We must revise the system now so that cost-conscious choices are encouraged and rewarded. This might be done within the present market-oriented system by relying more heavily on private health insurance. All citizens would be encouraged through tax incentives to purchase their own health care policies on the private market. Subsidies for those with low incomes would be provided in the form of vouchers or tax credits. Rather than expanding, Medicaid could be cut back to serve only as a safety net for individuals who cannot obtain private insurance because of a current illness or poor overall health. Cost-conscious consumers would encourage competition among insurers and providers to control costs. Cheaper policies with large deductibles might also help control costs by discouraging overuse of the system and rewarding 'healthy behaviour'.

But it is difficult to see how this consumer choice or market approach could solve the dual problems of access and cost. If the incentives to purchase insurance are large, they will greatly increase the budget deficit, offsetting any savings on Medicaid. If they are small, then many individuals and families will not purchase insurance or will purchase only limited coverage. When they need care it will be provided in the expensive emergency room setting, and the resulting cost-shifting will make insurance more expensive. Moreover, a more competitive free-market approach to insurance will intensify risk-pooling and the other underwriting practices that place coverage out of the reach of the people who need it most, throwing them back on the public sector. A private insurance solution might work if universal coverage could be achieved, but that would entail forcing individuals to purchase insurance and prohibiting discriminatory underwriting practices, neither of which would be attractive to civil libertarians or proponents of free markets. Finally, that competition and enlightened choice would control costs is dubious, since there seems little disincentive to develop and use increasingly expensive technology. As we have seen, competition in the health care industry tends to increase costs rather than diminish them.

Comprehensive Reform

The only effective way to resolve the current crisis in health care is to develop a system that features both universal coverage and budget limits. Universal coverage is necessary, not only because social justice requires it, but because it is the only way to stop cost-shifting. Budget limits are likewise necessary to develop and enforce cost control mechanisms and to maintain a predictable level of spending. The challenge is to design a programme that preserves the present system's quality of care, is congruent with basic American values of professional autonomy, market economics and consumer choice, and is achievable politically.

Socialised medicine, for example, in which physicians are salaried employees of a comprehensive, centrally budgeted and administered system, would provide the most reliable control of costs, but it is neither socially nor politically acceptable at the present time. The two most likely possibilities for attaining universal coverage and budget limits within a largely private system of health care delivery are mandated employment-based coverage and national health insurance.

Mandated Employer Coverage

The politically easiest means to universal coverage is some kind of mandated employer coverage since it would build on the present system and would preserve the private insurance sector. Most Americans receive their health insurance as an added benefit of employment. We tend to think of workplace coverage as part of the natural order of things, but our system actually took root during World War II, in large part because health benefits were exempt from wartime wage controls and thus could be offered (or demanded) in lieu of a rise in salary. After the war and the lifting of wage controls, the Internal Revenue Service ruled that the cost of health insurance was deductible from taxable income, and the popularity of employment-based coverage was more firmly established.[9]

One basic problem with this arrangement is that it has never covered everyone. Not all businesses offer health insurance, and the unemployed are left with inadequate public programmes such as Medicaid. Since it does form our largest base of coverage, however, it seems to many the easiest route to universal coverage. We could simply require every business to provide a minimum level of coverage, with defined benefits, to all its employees. Or we could adopt a so-called 'play or pay' system that would require businesses to provide the minimum level of coverage ('play') or pay into a public fund from which the uninsured would be covered. Small firms could pay the same rate as large ones, since the employees of many small firms would be combined to form large pools. The unemployed would still need to be covered, either by extending Medicaid or by including them in the large insurance pools with government subsidy.

The principal organised opposition to mandated coverage is from small businesses. Among firms with fewer than 10 employees, less than half offer health insurance.[10] Many fear that this added cost could not be absorbed, especially at current prices for small group coverage. For this reason mandated coverage must be accompanied by measures to reduce and control those prices. In addition to the pooling of small business employees we might do away with current practices of risk rating, that is, varying the cost of coverage according to the health status of the individual, and return to 'community rating', that is, basing a single price for a given level of coverage on the average health care costs for an entire community (not just healthy employed people). This would be good for the unemployed as well as for small businesses, since everyone could purchase coverage at the same rates. It would not be good, however, for large businesses, whose favoured rates would rise. More large firms could convert to self-insurance to preserve their advantage, skimming the cream and militating against the concept of community rating.

The most important factor in controlling the cost of health insurance, of course, is controlling the cost of health care. Spending is more difficult to control under a fragmented system of employer-based coverage and private insurance than under a single-payer programme of national health insurance. Nevertheless there are some successful models to examine. Hawaii has had a system of employer-based universal coverage for almost two decades. It combines mandated coverage with state subsidies and a state insurance pool for the unemployed. Insurers agreed to return to community ratings, and costs are controlled through annual fee-setting negotiations between insurers and providers. As a result, while everything else is more expensive in this island state, health insurance premiums in Hawaii are the lowest in the country.

Germany provides another example of a decentralised system with effective cost control. Most coverage is supplied by a multitude of regional, not-for-profit insurance organisations, known as 'sickness funds'. All employers are required to contribute at rates determined by the various funds. Fees are negotiated with physicians' associations, and rates are established with hospitals—the same daily rate for every patient, regardless of diagnosis. Under this system West Germany was able to restrict its growth in health care spending during the 1980s to the overall rate of growth of its gross domestic product.[11]

National Health Insurance

An important element of the cost of health care in the US is the expense of administering a diverse system of private health insurance. Under our present system insurance is provided by a multitude of companies competing on the private market, each with its own procedures and forms to complete for reimbursement. There are hundreds of kinds of policies and many levels of risk rating. Each company has its own administrative staff, and each provider must have several employees involved in keeping records and filling out various reimbursement forms. Add Medicare and Medicaid regulations and forms, and the result is that too much of our health care spending goes into administration and paperwork and too little into actual patient care. In 1987 the average overhead cost of private insurance carriers was 11.9% of premiums, compared with administrative costs of 3.2% for government programmes (primarily Medicare and Medicaid). Administrative costs for public and private programmes combined accounted for 5.1% of all health care expenditures in the US. By contrast the cost of administering the public health insurance programme in Canada was only 0.9%, and the figure for public and private programmes was 1.2%.[12]

How do the Canadians keep administrative costs so low? They have a single-payer system of national health insurance, covering all citizens equally, administered by the government and financed by taxes in lieu of insurance premiums. Consumers have freedom of choice among private practitioners, but as the single payer the government can set budgets and negotiate reasonable fees with providers. Seventy-three percent of all health spending is public (compared with 42% in the US). There is a small private insurance sector, but it is restricted by law to benefits not included in the public programme. Out-of-pocket payments are estimated to constitute 20% of all health expenditures (about the same as the US).[13] In addition to universal coverage, administrative efficiency and budgetary control, a system of national health insurance offers significant advantages. Since health insurance is uncoupled from employment, workers may change jobs without fear of losing their coverage. Dependents will remain insured if they become widowed or divorced from an employed spouse. Differential tax rates correlate coverage with ability to pay, avoiding inefficient and potentially humiliating means testing for public subsidies. Businesses need no longer purchase insurance in an unpredictable market and administer their own benefit programmes.

There are two large problems with instituting a system of national health insurance in the US: an immediate surge in unemployment and an uncertain 'utilisation response' to the new system. First, it is obvious that large numbers of insurance company employees (as well as billing clerks in hospitals and doctors' offices) would be out of work. Some would find employment with the new public programme, but not all, since the single-payer system would be more efficient. Since these are skilled workers most would find jobs sooner or later, but the immediate effect on an economy just beginning to recover from stagnation could be very serious. For these reasons we might have to phase in the new system, which would mean no effective cost controls for several more years. A new administration pledged to all three goals of economic growth, deficit reduction and immediate control of health care spending would face obvious political difficulties with a conversion to national health insurance. Although it seems to offer the best opportunity for long-term cost control and overall economic vitality, the short-term damage could be great.

The second serious concern is with the so-called utilisation response to the new system: would the response to free care be a surge in demand? If so, savings in administrative efficiency could be more than offset by increased consumption of services. One study estimates that universal access to free care would inflate expenditures by US$78.2 billion over 1991 levels while saving only US$46.8 billion in administrative costs.[14] This contradicts an earlier calculation that administrative savings would be sufficient to fund care for all the uninsured and underinsured.[15] All such predictions are generated from economic models that cannot adequately anticipate the complex behaviour of both patients and providers. We simply do not know what level of use to expect. Canada experienced no massive increase when its system was introduced, but as Barer and Evans aptly note, the US of 1994 is quite different from the Canada of 1967.

> A system that is awash with human and physical capacity and technical possibilities, and chafing under utilisation constraints that, while ineffective in aggregate, are still onerous and offensive, might very well respond to the extension of coverage with a significant increase in recommended diagnostic and therapeutic interventions. After all, one of the most common arguments for a universal system is to provide 'needed' care for those left out at present.[16]

Setting Priorities

Regardless of the direction health reform takes, moving from partial to universal coverage will be highly inflationary at the present rate of consumption. Reductions will be necessary somewhere—in fees, levels of coverage, or availability of services—to offset this inflationary pressure. The State of Oregon has developed a plan for extending coverage to all citizens while holding spending to current levels. It includes a play or pay requirement for employers, a high-risk pool funded from public and private sources, and a redistribution of Medicaid funds. The last feature has drawn the most attention. Under the proposed plan Medicaid eligibility would be extended to everyone below the federal poverty level. In order to cover more people with the same amount of money, fewer services will be included in the Medicare benefit package. A commission was created by the state legislature to develop, in the words of Senate Bill 27, the authorising legislation, 'a list of health services ranked by priority, from the most important to the least important, representing the comparative benefits of each service to the entire population to be served'.

Services would be included in the package as far down the list as budgeted funds would allow. The state has finally obtained a waiver from the federal government allowing it to use Medicaid funds in the proposed manner.

A national system with universal coverage would obviate the need for Oregon to implement its own programme, but its method of distributing scarce financial resources could be an important part of any national plan. While other schemes rely on some combination of fee negotiations, managed care, queues, or triage, Oregon plans to control costs by limiting services explicitly. Prioritising services could help determine minimum benefits for standardised insurance policies. Its most effective contribution, however, would be to a single-payer system, since it would allow periodic adjustments in coverage to enforce limits on spending. In combination with negotiated provider charges and limited deployment of expensive technology, it could be a powerful and flexible tool for both setting and enforcing a global budget.

Planning for the Future

Our Ageing Population

Lurking in the shadows of the debate on health care reform is a problem that threatens eventually to undermine any potential solution. Due in part to the post-war baby boom and subsequent steady decline in the birth rate, the average age of our population is steadily increasing. The trend will slow somewhat during the remainder of this decade, due to the relatively low birth rate during the Great Depression of the 1930s, but it will take a sharp upturn early in the next century. The first wave of the baby boom generation will reach retirement age (and eligibility for social security as well as Medicare) about 2011. By 2020, the elderly will account for approximately half of the nation's health care expenditure.[17] By 2040, the average age of the baby boom generation will be 85. After 85 average health costs increase dramatically.[18] Spending on hip fractures, for example, is projected to increase from US$1.6 billion in 1987 to as much as US$6 billion in 2040 (in constant 1987 dollars). More sobering still is the projection for the cost of care for demented individuals. The prevalence of dementia rises sharply after age 85; those who reach 85 have better than a one in four chance of becoming demented (this estimate may well be too low). In 2040 the cost of caring for demented patients alone is projected to be greater than the current federal deficit.[19]

Hip fractures and dementia are only two of the age-related conditions that require long-term care. Any comprehensive reform, indeed any reform of the health care system that hopes to provide access to basic care and control costs, must include long-term care. There are more residents of nursing homes than patients in hospitals or even available hospital beds.[20] Medicare does not include nursing home coverage, and the small number of private insurance policies available are of uncertain value. Nursing home stays are financed by personal savings and, when those are depleted, by Medicaid. Given current patterns of disability and nursing home use, the cost of long-term care could rise by 2040 to between US$84 and US$139 billion (in constant 1985 dollars).[19] Long-term care is not synonymous with nursing home care, though currently they are largely the same. Most of the millions of individuals who need long-term care neither want nor need nursing home placement, but their options are limited. Our challenge for the future is two-pronged: to provide less dispiriting and less expensive alternatives to nursing home care, and to integrate long-term care—both structurally and financially—into a comprehensive system of health care delivery.

Even without additional spending on long-term care, the share of the federal budget dedicated to pensions and health care is projected to increase from a current 40% to 60% by 2040. Without a sizeable tax increase, which seems unlikely, the money to fund entitlement programmes for the elderly may be taken from other sectors of the budget, such as education, public works and public assistance. If taxes were increased to cover such costs, there might be little remaining in the way of private savings to invest in the economy. Thus, a poorly educated, economically stagnant and stratified society could be the consequence of meeting all the health care demands of our ageing population.

Conclusion

Although an extension of employment-based health insurance would be the easier alternative to accomplish politically, a comprehensive system of national health insurance provides a better way to cope with the problems we face over the next 50 years. It seems clearly superior in three vital areas: coverage, efficiency and cost control. First, it is the only way to provide universal coverage that is the same for everybody. Other patchwork systems will have gaps and lapses in coverage and will include many different levels of coverage. A unified system will be easier for both patient and provider to understand and will promote social cohesion rather than division.

Second, a single-payer system will be more efficient. It will save overhead costs for both payer and provider and will eliminate the need for businesses to fund and administer employee health programmes. Businesses may still be taxed along with individuals to help fund the system, but the costs will be spread more evenly and will be predictable (ideally the cost to businesses should be no higher than those of their international competitors). The cost of regulation and review could also be greatly reduced. Without a single-payer system, considerable government regulation and oversight of the insurance industry will be necessary to achieve universal coverage at equitable rates. Managed care utilisation review could also be reduced under a programme of national health insurance. In addition, resources can be deployed more efficiently in a unified system than in a pluralistic one. Expensive equipment such as magnetic resonance imaging devices could be purchased to fill the needs of the population as a whole rather than the needs of competing organisations, thus avoiding unnecessary duplication of equipment and services.

Third, it is possible under a unified system to create budgets and to enforce them. The present fragmented system is structurally resistant to budgeting; there is no central authority to make a budget and few mechanisms for controlling spending. As we have seen, prioritising services would provide an additional measure of control and make adjustments easier. Resources could be developed and deployed with a view toward budgetary goals and limits. Long-term care and home health care could be integrated more easily into a comprehensive co-ordinated system. Thus a unified, single-payer plan would be more adaptable as we face the changing health care needs of an ageing population.

The task of health care reform is indeed daunting; for every two hands there seem to be three corks to hold under the water. Yet we must take immediate steps to control costs and expand coverage, and we must proceed with an eye toward the growing needs of an ageing population. The economic vitality as well as the moral character of our society are at stake as we prepare to enter the twenty-first century.

References

1. Jenks, S.F. and Schieber, G.J. (1991). Containing U.S. health care costs: what bullet to bite? *Health Care Financing Review 1991 Annual Supplement*, 1–12.
2. Sonnefeld, S.T., Waldo, R., Lemieu, J.A. and McKusic, D.R. (1991). Projections of national health expenditures through the year 2000. *Health Care Financing Review* **13** (1), 1–15.
3. A Report by the Families USA Foundation (1992). *Health Cost Squeeze on Older Americans*. Washington DC.
4. Meyer, H. (1993). Embattled insurers fight for survival. *American Medical News* **18**, 1.
5. Shelton, J.K. and Janosi, J.M. (1992). Unhealthy health care costs. *Journal of Medicine and Philosophy* **17**(1), 7–19.
6. Brown, M.L., Kessler, L.G. and Rueter, F.G. (1990). Is the supply of mammography machines outstripping need and demand? An economic analysis. *Annals of Internal Medicine* **113**(7), 547–552.
7. Shelton, J.K. and Janosi, J.M. (1992). Unhealthy health care costs. *Journal of Medicine and Philosophy* **17**, 7–19.
8. Webster, Jr. J.R. and Berdes, C. (1990). Ethics and economic realities. *Archives of Internal Medicine* **150**, 1795–1797.
9. Budetti, P. (1992). Universal health care coverage—pitfalls and promise of an employment-based approach. *Journal of Medicine and Philosophy* **17**, 21–32.
10. U.S. General Accounting Office (1990). *Health Insurance: Cost Increases Lead to Coverage Limitations and Cost Shifting*, Washington D.C. GAO/HRD 90–68.
11. Inglehart, J.K. (1991). Germany's health care system (first of two parts). *New England Journal of Medicine* **324**(7), 503–508.

12. Woolhander, S. and Himmelstein, D.U. (1991). The deteriorating administrative efficiency of the U.S. health care system. *New England Journal of Medicine* **324**(18), 1253–1258.
13. Schriber, G.J., Poullier, J.P. and Greenwald, L.M. (1992). U.S. health expenditure performance: an international comparison and data update. *Health Care Financing Review* **13**(4), 1–15.
14. Shields, J.F., Young, G.J. and Rubin, R.J. (1992). O Canada: do we expect too much from its health system? *Health Affairs* **11**(1), 7–20.
15. Woolhandler, S. and Himmelstein, D.U. (1988). Free care: a quantitative analysis of health and cost effects of a national health program for the United States. *International Journal of Health Services* **18**, 393–399.
16. Barer, M.L. and Evans, R.G. (1992). Interpreting Canada: models, mind-sets, and myths. *Health Affairs* **11**(1), 44–61.
17. U.S. Department of Health and Human Services (1988). *Health United States 1984*, Hyattsville, MD: U.S. Department of Health and Human Services, Publication PHS 88–1232, 1988:2.
18. Munoz, E., Rosner, F., Chalfin, D., Goldstein, J., Margolis, I. and Wise, L. (1989). Age resource consumption, and outcome for medical patients at an academic medical center. *Archives of Internal Medicine* **149**, 1946–1950.
19. Schneider, E.L. and Guralnik, J.M. (1990). The aging of America: impact on health care costs. *Journal of the American Medical Association* **263**(17), 2335–2340.
20. *Hospital Statistics*. (1987). American Hospital Association, Chicago.

Chapter 2

Oregon's Experiment

Michael Brannigan

La Roche College, Pittsburgh, USA

Background

With over 37 million Americans uninsured, Oregon's crisis is a microcosm of the nation's solemn failure in health care. In 1989, an estimated 400 000 Oregonians were uninsured. Of these 120 000 were unemployed, while the other 280 000 were in working households, unqualified for Medicaid—the public assistance programme for the poor. Medicaid eligibility is determined by each state, and Oregon had set its requirement at 58% below the federal poverty level. The federal poverty level for a single adult is an annual income of US$6620; for a family of four, it is US$12 000. Therefore, if that Oregon family makes over US$6960 per year, it becomes ineligible for public funding.[1]

The Medicaid predicament is heightened by other features, not least a conspicuous imbalance in funding within the programme. To illustrate, in 1988 although 70% of the nation's Medicaid population were children, they acquired only 12% of its funds. Also, although the poor are the intended recipients of Medicaid support, many of them do not benefit from its endowment. For instance, a leading group in the Medicaid programme is Aid to Families with Dependent Children (AFDC). Eligibility for AFDC continues to decrease, adversely affecting many children and single parents, especially women. In addition, even though the elderly and permanently disabled are in principle cared for under the federal Medicare programme, gaps in this programme necessitate supplementary Medicaid funding. (For a brief description of the distinction between Medicaid and Medicare, see Table 1.) Such discrepancies seem set to become yet more marked as average state spending on Medicaid rises: in 1991 spending stood at around 11% of state expenses, and it is estimated that this figure will grow to as much as 15% by 1995.[2]

While the nation floundered in its crisis, Oregon took steps early in the 1980s to confront squarely its difficulties (see Table 1). Issues of allocation were a

Reforming Health Care: The Philosophy and Practice of International Health Reform.
Edited by D. Seedhouse. © 1995 John Wiley & Sons Ltd.

Table 1 Chronology of key events in prioritisation

Key events

1982	Oregon Health Decisions created
October 11–12, 1984	First of three Citizens' Health Care Parliaments
September 1988	Oregon Medicaid Priority-Setting Project Health Services Commission established
April 1989	Oregon Basic Health Services Act approved by Oregon Senate
September 1989	HSC begins task of prioritisation
November 1989–February 1990	12 public hearings conducted
January–March 1990	OHD holds 47 community meetings
February 1990	Phone survey starts
May 2, 1990	HSC releases preliminary listing, *Cost/Utility Ratios Report*, with over 1600 items
May 1, 1991	First official Prioritised Health Services List; 709 line items; later funded through line 587
August 16, 1991	Oregon petitions federal government to waive 15 Medicaid requirements
April 22, 1992	Technical changes made in prioritised list
August 3, 1992	Denial of waiver request from Department of Health and Human Services
October 30, 1992	New prioritised list
November 13, 1992	Oregon resubmits waiver request to DHHS
December 4, 1992	Oregon Legislative Emergency Board funds revised list through line 568

Abbreviation

ADA	–	American Disabilities Act	MPP	–	Medicaid Priority-Setting Project
AFDC	–	Aid to Families with Dependent Children	OBHSA	–	Oregon Basic Health Services Act
DHHS	–	Department of Health and Human Services	OHD	–	Oregon Health Decisions
DRG	–	Diagnostic Related Groups	SB	–	Senate Bill
HCFA	–	Health Care Financing Administration	QALY	–	Quality Adjusted Life Year
HSC	–	Health Services Commission	QWB	–	Quality of Well-Being
MHCD	–	Mental Health and Chemical Dependency			

Medicare and Medicaid

These two federally-based programmes were established in the 1960s to serve the disadvantaged groups of the poor, elderly, and disabled. Due to the link between employment and health insurance, these groups were generally not covered. In effect, both programmes were a response to the evident failure of the market model of health care in the US.

Medicare is a federally supported insurance plan for those individuals who are over 65, with permanent disabilities, or with end-stage renal disease. It is an entitlement programme under federal guidelines, and citizens help subsidise it through federal taxes. Certain areas, however, are not covered under Medicare, such as long-term custodial care, prescription drugs, and eye and dental care. As stated earlier, much of the Medicaid funding is allocated to fill in some of these gaps.

Medicaid is a federal and state venture. It is not an entitlement plan since eligibility is not guaranteed. The federal government provides guidelines and contributes a share to each state's funding. However, states administer their programmes as well as set their own eligibility requirements. Eligibility therefore varies among states, and many have set their qualifications quite below the federal poverty level due to constrained state budgets.

dominant concern in the 1982 Governor's Conference on Health Care for the Medically Poor, and the Oregon Health Council established Oregon Health Decisions Inc. (OHD). OHD consequently played a major role in the prioritisation process since its objective was to stimulate public awareness of issues in bioethics, particularly in health care apportionment. Within 6 months during 1983 and 1984, OHD volunteers held nearly 300 meetings throughout the state, involving over 5000 Oregon citizens. An October 1984 Citizens' Health Care Parliament concluded with a report, *Society Must Decide*, behind which the sustaining consensus was that 'Health care rationing, cost containment, and health resource allocation were seen, first and foremost, as community matters'.[4] This view of health care as a community affair became a resounding premise throughout the later prioritisation plan. Setting the stage for the prospect of designing a health policy grounded upon community accord, Oregon's grass-roots style attracted the notice of other states, such as Maine, Wisconsin, California and Idaho.

In the following years, two more health care parliaments evoked further public discussions and recommendations for a more just health care system. Senator John Kitzhaber, a former emergency room physician and three times Oregon Senate President, assumed an energetic role in advocating universal access* and fair distribution of health services in the state.

In September 1988, Kitzhaber, OHD, John Golenski (President of the Bioethics Consulting Group, Berkeley) and others established the 'Oregon Medicaid Priority-Setting Project' (MPP). This undertaking concentrated on the principal groups of Medicaid beneficiaries (obstetrics and gynaecology, paediatrics, adult and geriatric) and ranked a variety of health care benefits from some general health service areas.

The legislature also established an 11-member Health Services Commission (HSC), whose goal was two-fold: expand Medicaid coverage and establish a list of prioritised health care services, to be periodically reviewed. Prioritisation recommendations would be made by the HSC to the legislature along with actuarial reports. If accepted, the state legislature (which meets for 6 months every 2 years) would then determine the level of funding for services for the next biennium, or 2-year session. This, in turn, would govern the range of health services to be offered.[2]

The effort to prioritise services is exceptional. Dwindling health care budgets are customarily reconciled either by lowering Medicaid eligibility (reducing access to health services), or by discounting reimbursements to providers. Oregon's strategy addresses its diminishing health care allowance by cutting those services which are lowest in priority. Therefore, this cut-off line defining the range of services 'floats' according to legislative determination of the state's financial health.

---

* 'Universal access' should not be equated with 'universal insurance scheme'. The majority of Oregonians, like most Americans, secure health insurance through a variety of means. The most common commercial plans are through employee benefits and private purchases. Medicaid and Medicare programmes are financed through public subsidies. In this report, 'universal access' refers to the access available to recipients of Medicaid funding.

The Oregon Basic Health Services Act of 1989

In April 1989, after months of legislative hearings and testimonies from various interest groups, the Oregon Basic Health Services Act (OBHSA) was passed by the Oregon Senate after overwhelming support in both houses. The act became law in July. It is a legislative package incorporating three separate, yet interrelated bills—Senate Bills (SB) 27, 534 and 935—which work together to provide access to basic health care services to nearly all of the uninsured (three more bills were passed in 1991).

SB27, the Basic Health Benefits Act, is the focus of our attention in this study. It is the cornerstone of the package and, undoubtedly, the most controversial. It seeks to extend Medicaid coverage to all uninsured Oregonians below the federal poverty level. While extending coverage, a prioritised list of services is determined by the Health Services Commission. This list ranks condition/treatment pairs (for example, biliary atresia/liver transplant, line number 92 in the most recent 30 October 1992 listing) according to the net-benefit of each, incorporating medical effectiveness and community values. This ranking assists the legislature's designation of the funding level, which will in turn demarcate a basic health care package for all citizens of Oregon.

The bill also specifies that prepaid managed care plans will be arranged with providers to help implement the project in an equitable fashion. In addition, physicians are required to inform patients of necessary procedures which will not be funded. Providers will have a 'liability shield', securing them from litigation in cases of not providing non-funded services below the line demarcated by legislation. (On the original May 1991 list of 709 line items, the line was drawn at 587. On the recently revised October 1992 list of 688 items, line 568 was the limit for state funding. This means that services below these lines, e.g. 588 and 569 respectively, are not required to be publicly funded under the Medicaid programme.) At the same time, there will be no decrease in payments to providers for their services.

This plan is a radical conversion from the current Medicaid programme, and its guidelines are notably different to current federal law. For example, it seeks to eliminate existing services mandated under Medicaid, which fall below the cut-off line. Therefore, Senate Bill 27 cannot be implemented without a federal waiver of certain programme requirements. At the same time, since the plan is considered a 'demonstration project' under Health Care Financing Administration rules, a federal waiver will allow the state to continue to receive current matching funds.[1]

SB 534, the State Health Risk Pool, intends to provide health care to those who are classified as uninsurable due to 'pre-existing medical conditions'. The state and private insurers will contribute to this 'risk pool', calculated to affect around 20 000 people.

SB 935, the Health Insurance Partnership Act, will require employers to offer the basic health benefit package from Senate Bill 27 to all full-time workers and their families. Employers and employees will share in the costs, the former contributing 75% and the latter 25%, with increased employee contributions for optional dependent coverage. Businesses will receive tax credits if they implement this before 1994. This proposal is estimated to affect around two-thirds of the uninsured in Oregon. (In 1991 Oregon passed Senate Bill 1076, which reinforces this bill.)

The fundamental axiom underlying the OBHSA is that all persons have a right to basic health care, that 'floor beneath which no person should fall'.[1] SB 27 commands our special attention. Its prioritised listing is a formative step requiring constant monitoring and reassessment. The Health Services Commission's 1991 report, *Prioritisation of Health Services*, describes the list as a 'prototype for ensuing development and refinement of the prioritisation process'.[1] SB 27 represents an impressive effort to rank health care services, and its methodology warrants further elaboration.

Subcommittees and Models

The 11-member Health Services Commission divided its task among five subcommittees. The task of the Social Values subcommittee was to gather and evaluate responses and concerns about health care values from the community. The Health Outcomes subcommittee was to obtain sufficient data from physicians and specialists concerning the medical effectiveness of treatments. The Mental Health and Chemical Dependency (MHCD) subcommittee's charge was to examine issues related to mental health, and to draft a prioritised catalogue of services which would eventually be integrated into the list of medical services. The first list would not include the MHCD ranking, but an integrated list would be a goal for the 1993–95 biennium. An Alternative Methodology subcommittee was later created to help reappraise and referee ranking mechanisms. The Ancillary Services subcommittee defined the kinds of auxiliary services integral to basic care that needed to be included in coverage, such as ambulatory, outpatient hospital, laboratory, prescription drugs, medical supplies, physical therapy, home health and hospice services.

The HSC's blueprint included linking the empirical data of medical effectiveness with community values, and there were no comparable models. The Oregon Medicaid Priority-Setting Project's earlier ranking was not specific enough. The HSC gave the core health systems of the UK, Germany, Sweden and Canada a 'cursory review', but it was felt that their systems were of little relevance to Oregon's purposes, and Alaska's procedure did not consider medical effectiveness and community values.[1] (It is interesting to note that at least three international visitors a month now come to Oregon to study the plan.) For a measurement tool, the HSC desired one which could feasibly include both data and values. Though no ideal method existed, Kaplan's Quality of Well-Being Scale (QWB) was selected because it appeared to encompass considerations of total health.[1]

Community Values

The Social Values subcommittee assumed the task of obtaining and appraising public values, in a well-coordinated effort through public hearings, community meetings and random telephone surveys.

Twelve public hearings were held in major cities, arranged through canvassing and media efforts along with Medicaid mailing announcements. The Oregon Health Action Council, an envoy for over 70 community organisations, provided additional support. Numbers at meetings ranged from 13 to 62, totalling over 1500 citizens. Various interest groups offered testimonies since the hearings were an occasion to discern public concerns, values and needs relevant to health care. The general conclusion was that preventive, MHCD and dental services should be a part of the standard benefits offered.[1]

The community meetings were organised and jointly conducted by OHD and the Senate Bill Community Meetings Advisory Committee. Strategies were devised to obtain an adequate cross-section of the populace, and 47 meetings in counties throughout the state were held. Attendance ranged from 3 to 120, averaging 20 per meeting. The total in attendance numbered 1048 in all.

The format of each community meeting was similar. Meetings usually lasted around 2 hours. Those who attended were seated at various tables, and questionnaires were distributed, describing condition and treatment situations such as:

A. Treatment of conditions which are fatal and cannot be cured. The treatment will not extend the person's life for more than 5 years.
C. Treatment for alcoholism or drug addiction.[1]

Each participant then rated each situation as: 'essential, very important or important'. This was followed by table discussions of the responses. These were in turn reported to the general assembly for a concluding discussion.

As a result of these meetings, 13 prominent values were highlighted, and, of these, the five most frequently discussed and apparently of highest concern were: prevention, quality of life, cost-effectiveness, ability to function and equity.[1] A demographic survey of the meetings was especially revealing. Over 69% of the participants were either health care or mental health workers; over 63% were women; an overwhelming number were insured (90.6%), and of these 4.4% were Medicaid recipients; 67% were college (university) graduates; 93% were white (the proportion of white adult Oregonians in the general population was 92%[1]; and 34% had annual household incomes of over US$50 000 (the average household income in the state was between US$24 000 and US$34 000).[1] While representation seemed adequate in some aspects, the degree of representation was a conspicuous concern on certain levels. While opinions were successfully gathered from those who attended, most of the participants were employed in a health care setting. Even more critically, low-income groups who would be the initially targeted population for Senate Bill 27 were drastically under-represented.[1] Nevertheless, the HSC's report did state that in those meetings where a higher percentage of uninsured attended, the values expressed were essentially the same. Still, OHD stressed the need for an all-out effort to elicit responses from the poor as a 'high priority'.[1]

A third part of this effort to establish community values was a random telephone survey of responses to questions concerning specific health states.

The survey instrument utilised Kaplan's QWB scale with slight modifications. Some 1001 telephone surveys were conducted through random digit dialing, and all state regions were proportionally accounted for. Respondents were first asked to assign a value from 0 to 100 for specific health states describing various combinations of functional impairments (affecting mobility, physical activity and social activity).

D. You can be taken anywhere, but have to be in bed or in a wheelchair controlled by someone else, need help to eat or go to the bathroom, but have no other health problems.

F. You cannot drive a car or use public transportation; you have to use a walker or wheelchair under your own control, and are limited in the recreational activities you may participate in. You have no other health problems.[1]

Next, respondents were asked to rate health states indicating major specific symptoms.

K. You can go anywhere and have no limitations on physical or other activity, but have stomach aches, vomiting or diarrhoea.

R. You can go anywhere and have no limitations on physical or other activity, but have trouble learning, remembering or thinking clearly.[1]

Responses to these situations were assigned weights and later applied to the health outcomes data provided by physicians and specialists.

Demographic data showed that women were over-represented while, as in the community meetings, those from low-income households were under-represented. As before, most of the respondents were white. Of the 1001 surveyed, 868 had private insurance, 80 were under Medicaid coverage, and at least 48 had no form of insurance whatsoever.[1] Of particular interest in the survey was that personal experience of a specific condition seemed to play a relevant role in perceiving the seriousness of the condition. That is, those who did not experience a condition tended to view that condition as more severe than those who had had some experience.

Health Outcomes Assessment

Establishing the overall medical outcome of treatments for specific conditions involved an intricate process. Not only was there an absence of previous models, but a review of the research literature indicated inconclusive reports as well as insufficient data. Testimony had to be obtained from physicians, particularly from specialty organisations.

Initially, cost-effectiveness was a primary factor, but this was eventually replaced by overall net-benefit. This net-benefit was determined by calculating the Quality of Well-Being (QWB) with the proposed treatment minus the QWB without the treatment. Relevant factors included in this formula were: information on the effectiveness of treatment, using the median age at onset for specific conditions, estimating the duration of treatment benefits, and considering total treatment costs. The Commission report illustrated this net-benefit formula using the condition of acute myocardial infarction.

1. Information was gathered about the effectiveness of treating heart attacks; both treatment and non-treatment probabilities were established.
2. The median age at onset of this condition is 46 years (the middle of the midpoint cohort).
3. The duration of benefit was established by subtracting the onset age from life-expectancy ($75 - 46 = 29$ years).
4. Total treatment costs were factored in.
5. A QWB score was then assigned to both treatment and non-treatment states.
6. The net benefit was that difference between QWB with treatment minus QWB without treatment. In the case of acute myocardial infarction, the QWB with treatment was clearly higher than that without treatment.[1]

Within this calculation, health states were essentially defined in three ways: the probability of mortality, the likelihood of a return to an asymptomatic state (the state of health 'before the onset of the condition being treated'), and degrees of morbidity, or 'significant residual effects' from the treatment 'comprised of symptoms and functional impairments'. This intricate process of obtaining health outcomes provided the empirical base for prioritisation.[1]

Prioritisation

The ranking procedure can be abridged by viewing it, as the HSC report suggests, in three distinct stages.

Step 1. Seventeen general categories were developed and differentiated according to the nature of the conditions (whether acute or chronic, fatal or non-fatal; according to the degree of morbidity, and so on). Criteria were then designed to rank these categories, and weights were allotted to each criteria.

Value to society:	weight of 40
Value to the individual at risk:	weight of 20
Essential to basic care:	weight of 40

Each category was then ranked in order of importance according to these three criteria. Here is a selection from the final ranking of categories followed by illustrative examples:

1. *Acute Fatal*, treatment prevents death with full recovery: appendectomy for appendicitis; repair of deep, open wound in neck; medical therapy for myocarditis.
2. *Maternal Care*, including most disorders of the newborn: obstetric care for pregnancy.
5. *Chronic Fatal*, treatment improves life span and quality of life: medical therapy for Type 1 diabetes mellitus; medical and surgical treatment for

treatable cancer of the uterus; medical therapy for asthma.

7. *Comfort Care*: palliative therapy for conditions in which death is imminent.[1]

According to their ranking, categories were grouped as being essential, very important, or important to certain individuals:

Categories 1–9:   essential
Categories 10–13:   very important
Categories 14–17:   important to certain individuals.[3]

Step 2. Condition/treatment pairs were then assigned to appropriate categories. Consequently, each pair was ranked using a net-benefit analysis. Outcome data were provided by specialists, who assessed degrees of morbidity and quality of life of designated symptoms and functional impairment. The net-benefit score for each condition/treatment pair determined their rank within each category, resulting in a draft list of prioritised services.

Step 3. The HSC made adjustments to this draft list of ranked services. This was to ensure the proper placement of items 'out-of-position', and to maintain consistency with community values. The HSC used a 'reasonableness' standard in their adjustments, balancing six components: 'public health impact, cost of medical treatment, incidence of condition, effectiveness of treatment, social costs and cost of non-treatment'. The commissioners also explained that 'it was not reasonable—logically or economically—to rank preventable or readily treatable conditions in relatively unfavourable positions. In other words, where severe or exacerbated conditions were ranked in a relatively favourable position compared to prevention of disease, disability or exacerbation, these occurrences were reversed'.[1]

The first official prioritisation list, containing 709 items, was produced in May 1991. A sample of the first page of the list is given in Table 2. Its coding and classification can be illustrated with item 587, oesophagitis (determined as the cut-off point for funding on this list).*

Diagnosis: Oesophagitis
Treatment: Medical therapy
    ICD–9:   530.1
      CPT: 90000–99999
      Line: 587   Category: 13.[1]

---

* ICD–9 refers to the *International Classification of Diseases* (9th edn) code number which describes the condition.

   CPT refers to the *Physician's Current Procedural Terminology* to indicate numeric codes which describe the treatment procedure(s) for the condition.

   The line number refers to the order assigned to this condition/treatment pair in the prioritisation. *Line item 1 is most essential while item 709 is least essential.*

   The Category number refers to the general category which was ranked in the first stage of the prioritisation process above. Category 1 is most important while category 17 is least important. (This category feature was deleted from the revised list of October 1992.)

   Note that not all condition/treatment pairs are grouped together according to categories due to the Commission's final adjustments.

Table 2   Prioritised Health Services list of 1 May 1991

Diagnosis:	Pneumococcal pneumonia, other bacterial pneumonia, bronchopneumonia, influenza with pneumonia
Treatment:	Medical therapy
ICD–9:	020.3–5, 022.1, 073, 466, 481–483, 485–486, 487.1
CPT:	90000–99999
Line:	1 Category: 1
Diagnosis:	Tuberculosis
Treatment:	Medical therapy
ICD–9:	010–012
CPT:	90000–99999
Line:	2 Category: 5
Diagnosis:	Peritonitis
Treatment:	Medical and surgical treatment
ICD–9:	567
CPT:	90000–99999
Line:	3 Category: 1
Diagnosis:	Foreign body in pharynx, larynx, trachea, bronchus and oesophagus
Treatment:	Removal of foreign body
ICD–9:	933.0–.1, 934.0–.1, 935.1
CPT:	31635, 40804
Line:	4 Category: 1
Diagnosis:	Appendicitis
Treatment:	Appendectomy
ICD–9:	540–543
CPT:	44950, 44900, 44960
Line:	5 Category: 1
Diagnosis:	Ruptured intestine
Treatment:	Repair
ICD–9:	569.3
CPT:	44600–10
Line:	6 Category: 1
Diagnosis:	Hernia with obstruction and/or gangrene
Treatment:	Repair
ICD–9:	550.0–.1, 551–552
CPT:	39502–41, 443330–31, 43885, 44050, 44346, 49500–611, 49500–611, 49500–11, 49000, 51500, 55540
Line:	7 Category: 1

Table 2   (*continued*)

Diagnosis:	Group syndrome, acute laryngotracheitis
Treatment:	Medical therapy, intubation, tracheotomy
ICD–9:	464.0–.5
CPT:	90000–99999, 31500, 31600
Line:	8 Category: 1
Diagnosis:	Acute orbital cellulitis
Treatment:	Medical therapy
ICD–9:	376.0
CPT:	90000–99999
Line:	9 Category: 1
Diagnosis:	Ectopic pregnancy
Treatment:	Surgery
ICD–9:	633
CPT:	58700, 587200, 58770, 58980, 59135
Line:	10 Category: 1
Diagnosis:	Injury to major blood vessels of upper extremity
Treatment:	Ligation
ICD–9:	903
CPT:	37618
Line:	11 Category: 1
Diagnosis:	Ruptured spleen
Treatment:	Repair/splenectomy/incision
ICD–9:	865.04
CPT:	38100, 49000, 38115
Line:	12 Category: 1

The report claimed that the two most important considerations in the official May 1991 listing were ranked categorisation and net benefit. Overall, this was an elaborate, systematic effort at a just method for prioritising health services within a limited budget.

After the list, accompanied by an actuarial analysis, was formally adopted, the Oregon legislation then determined the cut-off line for funding. As we stated above, this first list was to be funded through line 587 (items falling on either side of the cut-off line for the May 1991 list are displayed in Table 4). However, as was mentioned earlier, the implementation of the list requires particular Medicaid waivers from the HCFA. It needs to be stressed that Medicaid is not exclusively a state programme. A substantial portion of the funding is allocated by the federal government. Oregon's project needs to be envisioned in broader political strokes. Even though Oregon's legislation sets the eligibility requirements and ultimately defines the basic health care package, the full activation of the Oregon plan is contingent upon the federal response. As of this writing, rationing is in effect with respect to Senate Bills

Table 3   Prioritised list of health services 30 October 1992

Diagnosis:	Severe/moderate head injury: haematoma/oedema with loss of consciousness
Treatment:	Medical and surgical treatment
ICD–9:	850.1–850.5, 851.02–851.02–851.06, 851.1, 851.22–851.26, 851.3851.42–851.46, 851.5, 851.62–851.66, 851.7.851.82–851.86, 851.9
CPT:	61108, 61313–61315, 62140–62141
Line:	1
Diagnosis:	Insulin-dependent diabetes mellitus
Treatment:	Medical therapy
ICD–9:	250.01, 250.1–250.3, 250.6, 251–3, 775.1
CPT:	11400–11402, 11420, 90000–99999
Line:	2
Diagnosis:	Peritonitis
Treatment:	Medical and surgical treatment
ICD–9:	567, 777.6
CPT:	11400–11402, 11420, 90000–99999
Line:	3
Diagnosis:	Acute glomerulonephritis: with lesion or rapidly progressive glomerulonephritis
Treatment:	Medical therapy including analysis
ICD–9:	580.4
CPT:	90000–99999
Line:	4
Diagnosis:	Patent ductus arteriosus
Treatment:	Ligation
ICD–9:	747.0
CPT:	33820–33822
Line:	5
Diagnosis:	Pneumothorax and haemothorax
Treatment:	TUVE thoracostomy/thoracotomy, medical therapy
ICD–9:	511.8, 512, 860
CPT:	32020, 32500, 90000–99999
Line:	6
Diagnosis:	Hernia with obstruction and/or gangrene
Treatment:	Repair
ICD–9:	550.0–550.1, 551–552
CPT:	39502–39541, 43330–43331, 43885, 44050, 44346, 49500–49611, 51500, 55540
Line:	7

Table 3   *(continued)*

Diagnosis:	Appendicitis
Treatment:	Appendectomy
ICD–9:	540–543
CPT:	44900, 44950, 44960
Line:	8
Diagnosis:	Addison's disease
Treatment:	Medical therapy
ICD–9:	255.4, 255.5
CPT:	90000–99999
Line:	9

534, 935 and 1076, that is, from private and employment insurers. However, SB 27 is still waiting for Medicaid waivers before its publicly funded rationing plan can be implemented.

Events after the May 1991 List

In April 1992, coding errors along with improvements in some medical technologies required technical changes to the first list. The new list still contained 709 items, and funding was still set at item 587. Early on, prospects for legislative approval of the waiver request seemed optimistic, despite opposition from Senators Albert Gore Jr and Henry Waxman. In August 1992, a surprising turn of events came about when Oregon's request for Medicaid waivers was denied. The Department of Health and Human Services (DHHS) Secretary Louis Sullivan's memorandum to the Oregon HSC disclosed that its grounds for rejection centred around the American Disabilities Act (ADA). Specific elements in the Oregon proposal were in potential violation of basic ADA tenets and thereby appeared to discriminate against the disabled. Two components in particular were singled out: the QWB scale used in the telephone surveys, and the final 'hand adjustments' made by members of the HSC.

The HSC essentially disagreed with the DHHS judgement. Despite this, and in view of the fact that SB 27 could only be set in motion with federal waivers, the HSC worked on revising the original list in order to address possible areas of discrimination. Since the DHHS claimed that the telephone survey weights 'gave the perception that Oregon valued the quality of life of a person without disabilities above that of a person with disabilities', the HSC withdrew the data from the telephone survey as well as 'quality of life' references. The health outcomes database of symptom descriptors and numeric codes, as well as the numeric weights for functional impairments were deleted. At the same time, the methodology was simplified. Net benefit and medical effectiveness were arrived at by considering, in order, the treatment's ability to: (1) maintain life, (2) restore one to an asymptomatic state, (3) be cost-effective, and (4) be consistent with community values.[6]

Table 4   Some condition/treatment items on both sides of the cut-off line (line 587) on the May 1991 prioritisation list

Diagnosis:	Disorders of cervical region
Treatment:	Cervical laminectomy, medical therapy
ICD–9:	721.0, 722.4, 722.81, 723
CPT:	63250, 63265, 63270, 63275, 63280, 63285, 63001, 63015, 63020, 63035–40, 63045, 63048, 63075–76, 63081–82, 63300, 63304, 63170,–72, 63180–82, 63194, 63196, 63198, 90000–99999
Line:	583 Category: 13
Diagnosis:	Erythematous conditions: toxic, nodosum, rosacea, lupus
Treatment:	Medical therapy
ICD–9:	695.0, 695.2–.9
CPT:	90000–99999, 11100–11101
Line:	584 Category: 13
Diagnosis:	Plantar fascial fibromatosis
Treatment:	Medical therapy
ICD–9:	728.71
CPT:	90000–99999
Line:	585 Category: 13
Diagnosis:	Spondylosis and other chronic disorders of back
Treatment:	Medical and surgical treatment
ICD–9:	720, 721.2–.5 721.7, 721.9, 722.3–.5, 722.7–.9, 723.0, 724, 738.4, 756.11, 847
CPT:	22100, 22105, 22110, 22140–230, 22548–54, 22590–650, 22820–99, 62284, 62290–1, 63001–48, 63075–8, 63081–2, 63085–8, 63090–1, 63300–4, 90000–99999
Line:	586 Category: 13
Diagnosis:	Oesophagitis
Treatment:	Medical therapy
ICD–9:	530.1
CPT:	90000–99999
Line:	587 Category: 13
Diagnosis:	Intervertebral disc disorders
Treatment:	Thoracic–lumbar laminectomy, medical therapy
ICD–9:	722.0–1, 722.7, 952.1–9
CPT:	63003, 63005, 63016, 63017, 63030–31, 63035, 63042, 63046–48, 63056–57, 63064, 63066, 63077–78, 63085–91, 63170, 63173, 90000–99999
Line:	588 Category: 13
Diagnosis:	Chronic prostatitis, other disorders of prostate
Treatment:	Medical therapy
ICD–9:	601.1, 602
CPT:	90000–99999
Line:	589 Category: 13

Table 4   (*continued*)

Diagnosis:	Chronic cystitis
Treatment:	Medical therapy
ICD–9:	595.1–595.3
CPT:	90000–99999
Line:	590 Category: 13
Diagnosis:	Impetigo herpetiformis and subcorneal postular dermatosis
Treatment:	Medical therapy
ICD–9:	694.0–3
CPT:	90000–99999
Line:	591 Category: 13

The principal changes in the list were: (1) the deletion of category numbers; (2) the inclusion of neuromuscular dysfunction encompassing several conditions grouped together within the same item, line 152 (including cerebral palsy, amyotrophic lateral sclerosis, and anencephaly); (3) the exclusion of end-stage human immunodeficiency virus (HIV) infection so that various HIV conditions and treatment were assigned to several items; (4) blending all liver cirrhosis/liver transplants into one item (line 132); (5) consolidating treatments for all babies under 2500 grams into one item (line 40). These accomodations addressed likely areas of sensitivity of the ADA.

The HSC made its final judgement with input from representatives of disability groups. After a public meeting to discuss the changes, and confident that the revised list fairly embodied both medical effectiveness and community values, the HSC sanctioned the new list on 30 October 1992. The total number of items on the revised list was reduced from 709 to 688. (A sample of the first page of the revised list is given in Table 3.) In early December, the Oregon legislature approved the revised list and funded services through line 568. Here are two examples of items not funded in this revised list, lines 642 and 670, acute viral hepatitis and cancer with less than a 5% 5-year survival.

Diagnosis:	Acute viral hepatitis
Treatment:	Medical therapy
ICD–9:	070
CPT:	90000–99999
Line:	642

Diagnosis:	Cancer of various sites with distant metastases where treatment will not result in a 5% 5-year survival
Treatment:	Medical and surgical treatment
ICD–9:	140–198
CPT:	11600–11646, 38720–38724, 41110–41114, 41130, 42120, 42842–42845, 42880, 44131, 47610, 47420–47440, 58951, 61500, 61510, 61518–61521, 61546–61548, 90000–99999.
Line:	670[6]

Table 5 Some condition/treatment items on both sides of the cut-off line (line 568) on the revised October 1992 prioritisation list. Condition/treatment pairs below line 568 are not to be publicly funded (if waiver request is granted)

Diagnosis:	Congenital dislocation of knee, genu varum and valgum (acquired), congenital bowing of femur, tibia and fibula, genu recurvatum (acquired), congenital genu recurvatum long bones of legs, congenital deformities of knee
Treatment:	Osteotomy
ICD–9:	736.4, 754.40–754.43, 755.64
CPT:	27455, 27448–27450
Line:	564
Diagnosis:	Lesion of plantar nerve
Treatment:	Medical therapy, excision
ICD–9:	355.6
CPT:	28080, 90000, 99999
Line:	565
Diagnosis:	Bone spur
Treatment:	Ostectomy
ICD–9:	726.91
CPT:	28119, 28899
Line:	566
Diagnosis:	Peripheral nerve injury with open wound
Treatment:	Neuroplasty
ICD–9:	953.4–953.9, 954–956, 957.9
CPT:	64702–64727, 64732–64792, 64830–64876
Line:	567
Diagnosis:	Peripheral nerve disorders (non-injury)
Treatment:	Neuroplasty
ICD–9:	353.0–353.4, 354.1, 354.9, 355.0, 350.2, 355.6, 355.8
CPT:	64702–64727, 64774–64792
Line:	568
Diagnosis:	Disorders of sweat glands
Treatment:	Medical therapy
ICD–9:	705.0, 705.81, 705.89, 705.9, 780.8
CPT:	90000–99999
Line:	569
Diagnosis:	Disorders of soft tissue
Treatment:	Medical therapy
ICD–9:	729
CPT:	90000–99999
Line:	570 Category: 13

Table 5   *(continued)*

Diagnosis:	Disorders of synovium, tendon and bursa
Treatment:	Medical therapy
ICD–9:	727.2–727.3
CPT:	90000–99999
Line:	571
Diagnosis:	Non-inflammatory disorders of cervix
Treatment:	Medical therapy
ICD–9:	622.4, 622.6–622.9, 624.2, 624.6–624.9
CPT:	90000–99999
Line:	572

(A listing of some services above and below the cut-off line for the October 1992 list is given in Table 5.) Oregon resubmitted its waiver request and, at the time this article was first written, anticipated a more positive response from the DHHS.

Plan Finally Approved

The Oregon plan was finally approved by the Clinton Administration through an affirmative ruling by the Secretary of Health and Human Services, Donna Shalala, on 19 March 1993. Twenty-nine conditions were stipulated, 26 dealing with formalisation of the waiver process. Three directly impact upon the substance of the prioritised listing. These three contingencies are as follows. First, the listing needs to be redone without symptomatology as a formal criterion. This leaves the major criteria in the listing as: death, cost, and HSC judgement. This has only produced some minor changes. Second, the value of 'infertility', considered a disability, is to be removed. Four lines were effected. Third, an 800 (toll free) number is to be developed for call-in lines from physicians. In April 1993, the number of lines in the listing was extended to 696, with the cut-off line resting at line number 565. This listing stayed the same in January 1994 with the same cut-off line. In summary, this has not produced any major changes in the listing, according to Paige Sipes-Metzler, Executive Director of the Oregon HSC. Given these contingencies the plan actually went into effect 1 February 1994. Within the next five years, the uninsured will be gradually phased into the plan. As of April 1994, there were over 35 220 enrollees, the majority of whom are families.

Ethical Issues

Although still fresh, Oregon's rationing scheme has already produced much friction. In the following précis of the more prominent arguments in the debate,

I have arranged positions in favour of the prioritisation plan into three areas:

1. Arguments centring around context.
2. Critiques of idealism.
3. Arguments endorsing the process.

Objections to the scheme are grouped into three types:

1. Objections to the plan's scope or content.
2. Objections to its process.
3. Objections based on implications of the plan.

Supporting Testimonies

Advocates for the project often emphasise the political and long-range context in which the OBHSA should be perceived and understood. The prioritisation plan is part of a total design to enhance access to health care for all Oregonians. It needs to be viewed as part of a package consisting of distinct bills oriented toward its foremost goal which is not prioritisation for targeted groups of poor, but a major health care system reform affecting all parties. For instance, the bills working in tandem would eventually establish an integration of Medicaid and Medicare in its coverage of a long-term care insurance programme. Even though critics allege unfair exemptions such as for the elderly, advocates claim that, in the long term, all parties, including the elderly, would be benefited.[7] Alexander Capron reports further that in 1993, it is projected that 'SB 27 will encompass Medicaid-eligible elderly, disabled, and foster-care patients, thereby greatly expanding the pool of funds available'.[8] Critics often misconstrue this proper context by treating the list of items as the final product. Instead, it is meant to begin a long process of debate, reassessment and negotiation with the ultimate political goal of a national system of universal health care.

An essential ingredient in this wider context is Oregon's bold attempt to define a basic health care package. If it successfully defines and implements this, then it is on its way toward eliminating wasteful spending on ineffective procedures. Oregon has already proved its willingness to make more efficient use of its drastically limited Medicaid funding by shifting into prepaid contracts with managed care programmes.[8] These earlier attempts at cost-effectiveness need to accompany how we perceive its present, long-range efforts.

Given this, Oregon's project is a provocative state experiment from which to absorb and learn. Its efforts will be monitored by other states, and the strengths and weaknesses of its process will be a constructive guide for programmes aiming for universalised forms of health care. Oregon's initiative is a systematic and creative first step in this direction, a corrective to an urgent situation, state and nationwide.

Critics respond that, if we are to conceive of the Oregon plan as a state experiment, then with what criteria can we properly evaluate its progress, particularly in view of the absence of any earlier 'needs assessment'? Dougherty, for instance, has stressed that clear standards for evaluation and monitoring need to be set.[7]

Advocates often accuse the plan's detractors of unfair idealism. They claim that critics expend energies pointing out flaws in Oregon's project with arguments that are 'disengaged from reality', and neglect or underestimate serious flaws in the current system. In Oregon, the health status of the poor continues to decline. And it is a shameful fact that hundreds of thousands in Oregon and tens of millions in the country remain uninsured. Supporters feel that while critics argue against the explicit rationing scheme of Oregon, they fail to heed sufficiently the implicit rationing which already occurs in various forms. Eligibility for Medicaid recipients in the state is set at 58% of the federal poverty level. This is rationing based upon income. John Golenski terms it 'rationing by non-access'.[quoted in 10] Furthermore, these ineligibles, the working uninsured, most of whom consist of families with children, subsidise coverage for others through a portion of their taxes, which contribute to state and federal expenditures.[7] In addition, the provision of charity health care to the uninsured has led to increased medical rates, resulting in a form of 'cost-shifting', whereby consumers, and especially employers, pay escalating fees for their own non-charity medical services.[1]

These harsh realities exist within the broader contours of the prevailing system's 'bias toward high-cost, high-technology medical care'.[13] Kitzhaber echoes this sentiment, and cites explicit failures in Oregon's Medicaid pattern. First, due to an overemphasis upon health care as an end in itself rather than as a means to an end, the present system wrongly assumes that access necessarily produces equitable results. Second, there is the precarious misconception on the part of the policy-makers that 'all health services are equal'. Third, governmental practice reveals a lack of commitment to entitlement based upon need. Next, Medicare entitlements exist but not so with Medicaid. Current inequities are exacerbated and tax credits generally privilege the wealthy and the middle class. Finally, current political economic and social realities appear to militate against an equitable system of health care. Within a strong capitalistic framework, individuals will still purchase what they can afford in an open market. Americans pay lip service to the need for national health insurance, as they remain reluctant to dole out additional taxes and endure necessary cutbacks.[7]

On the other hand, opponents acknowledge inequities, yet they question whether Oregon's approach is any less unfair. Objecting to the plan does not suggest an endorsement of the current situation. Other avenues to universal access exist and need to be explored.[7]

Supporters concede to weaknesses in the prioritisation plan, but declare that the vital question is whether the Oregon plan is better than the status quo. They argue that the 'worst off' in our current health system, namely, the uninsured and unemployed, stand to gain from the plan on two counts: not only will they gain access to health care, but more people will be able to receive more medically effective treatment, since, by eliminating services that are least beneficial, coverage is extended to those of better net-gain.[7]

Oregon's controversial process, or methodology, continues to be justified by supporters as both comprehensive and fair. Gathering and combining clinical data and public values was effectively accomplished. Acquiring a sense of community values was an especially innovative enterprise. The sincere and open manner in which discussions transpired has been hailed as an 'exercise in American democracy'.[2] The evolution of OHD revealed ongoing efforts to involve the community in matters of critical concern. Key phases within the process were tempered by community values, contributing to the single aim of a quality health care system. The public hearings, community meetings, and phone surveys demonstrate the vital aspect of public accountability. These public meetings can be regarded as an animating 'goad to the public'. The well-being of the immediate target of the prioritisation plan, Medicaid recipients and the uninsured, depends in good measure upon the public's willingness to contribute their fair share. Public meetings are worthwhile in making more visible the current system's implicit rationing and its inequities.[11]

Defenders of the plan single out several positive methodological attributes. For one, the process contains elemental 'safeguards'. The HSC's judgements are balanced by input from community and specialists. In addition to this internal check-and-balance, third-party review by the DHHS provides external scrutiny.[13] Plus, the HSC's use of general health state categories makes better sense than having more constricted ones. This permits a more realistic accommodation of individual condition/treatment pairs. Moreover, the use of Quality Adjusted Life Years (QALYs) remains a useful technique since it integrates quality of life concerns with duration of benefits. In this respect, the Oregon plan makes 'its greatest methodological contribution to the goal of setting health care priorities'.[5]

Hadorn distinguishes between employing quality of life gauges in a discriminatory fashion and their justifiable use by Oregon. If the quality of life measurement centres on a fixed point in time for a specific patient aside from treatment concerns, the potential for discrimination exists. Oregon's method, however, is to evaluate the change that would likely occur due to treatment over a period of time. 'At the same time, the potential for discrimination is eliminated because treatments for handicapped or "poor quality of life" patients are evaluated on the same basis as are treatments for everyone else. It is the *change* in quality of life, or net benefit, realised from a *treatment* that matters, not the *point-in-time* quality of life of a *patient*'.[5] In addition, economic concerns were not major factors in the official listings. The critical consideration was that of quality of life, an issue often raised in the earlier meetings held by OHD throughout the community.

Opposing Arguments

Oregon's plan aims to help the uninsured, most of whom are below the federal poverty level. Yet opponents declare that its scope is blatantly unfair, particularly for 'poor mothers and children'. Under the current system, those in AFDC have access to the same benefits as the more affluent. Under Oregon's plan, this same group will have benefits reduced in order to expand coverage.[14] Burdens will not be equitably shared, since few burdens will be carried by those above the federal poverty level, and providers will continue to benefit since there is no reduction in reimbursements. This constitutes one of the most plaguing issues in Oregon's scheme.

In response, supporters declare that the 'worst off' under the present system are not the AFDC recipients, but those without any insurance whatsoever. They claim that the plan does help these worst off, while the burdens are shared. SB 935 legislates that employers finance most of the costs, while SB 534 stipulates subsidisation by both private insurers and the state for a risk pool fund.[7] Moreover, the rationale for exempting the elderly lies in the fact that most of the services required for the elderly are social, and most of their medical services are Medicare-covered. Including the elderly at this point would therefore appear to be beyond the prerogatives of the Medicaid programme.[13]

Nevertheless, opponents retort, targeting the poor is still unfair, for it singles out a vulnerable group and threatens social integrity. A line-drawing prioritisation process will lead to social line-drawing.[7] Some critics add that the real rationale for the plan is more political than altruistic, a strategy to 'gain political leverage over costly, marginal, mandated services' insisted upon by provider lobbies.[14]

The process of prioritisation has drawn rancour due to its very idea, some averring that rationing is inherently immoral and brings about an unjust distribution of services.[7] Furthermore, critics argue that Oregon does not even deserve to engage in the process of ranking services, because it has not engineered sufficient preliminary efforts to excise wasteful spending. The state did not exhaust other means to enhance access such as raising taxes or shifting funds from other programmes. And it has not substantially added funds to its Medicaid programme. In Medicaid spending, it ranks 46th in the nation.[15]

Opponents add that, if the Oregon plan is to be recognised as an experiment, or 'demonstration project', the glaring under-representation of the targeted poor precludes any possibility of their valid consent.

The rejoinder to this asks: with what particular mechanisms can consent be adequately obtained? In addition, since Medicaid funding is essentially provided from public resources, what about expanding the scope of consent?[18] Capron attaches a further point when he claims that Oregon's initiative is strictly a 'social policy experiment', and therefore is generally exempted from such consent requirement.[8]

The idea and process of gathering a community consensus has generated alarm from the critics. To begin with, to what extent *should* the public be involved in such technical matters as prioritising health care services and in influencing public policy decisions? Public wisdom provides an insecure basis for a system of quality health care. Along the same lines, how can individuals evaluate poor health states which they have not even experienced? This is a critical issue, and becomes a sore point in the subsequent waiver rejection. Furthermore, not only were the targeted groups not fairly represented, but most of the participants in the community meetings were college-educated, somewhat affluent, associated with health professions, and white. And this raises another concern. By what suitable standards can community values be ranked? In addition, some values are vague while others are more medical than ethical, such as prevention and MHCD.[7] Finally, a frequent criticism of this part of the process is the vague nature of the relationship between community values and the final ranking made by the HSC. It remains unclear just how these public values are to act as a 'check' on medical outcomes and QWB measurements.[7]

Critics also suspect the validity of the outcomes assessment methodology. For instance, co-morbidity states are not measured, an important neglect since the presence of other conditions can often affect the medical outcomes of treatments. In addition, there is a lack of sufficient, current medical-effectiveness data. Furthermore, condensing over 10 000 specific health conditions into viable categories may suggest similarities among conditions and treatment modalities where none exist.[14] Moreover, the language in the questionnaires (for example, the phrase 'trouble talking') is at best vague, and the assignment of negative numerical scores to certain illness states is at times puzzling. Rating responses over the phone seems especially troublesome.[5]

The use of QALYs as a factor in the ranking process disturbs critics. As a component in the QWB scale, its value as a gauge has been questioned on a number of counts: its suggestion that quality of life can be quantified, its utilitarian presuppositions, its assumption of the compatibility of equity and efficiency, an apparent tyranny of communal preferences over individual interest, the premise that older and sicker patients stand to gain less from treatments, and finally its assumption that physicians will not be affected in their role as patient advocates.[16] A cold, utilitarian calculus which subsumes all interests solely within a communal framework draws much criticism. And evaluating the quality of life of others is inherently dangerous. On a more phenomenological level, what is the relationship between an objective measurement of quality of life, such as QALYs and QWB scale, and a subjective perception of quality of life?

In this context, since Oregon's project evidently regards 'basic care' as that which is 'morally prior', certain assumptions are morally questionable. Robert Veatch argues that this is particularly the case if cost considerations are factored into the notion of 'basic', a term filled with ambiguities.[9] Rudolf Klein concludes that the presence of assumptions which may be morally suspect in both defining and rationing a package of health services entitles Oregon's plan to more of a 'warning rather than offering a model for import into Britain'.[17]

Many fear the implications of prioritisation, especially its effect upon the physician/patient relationship. Critics claim that Oregon's initiative reinforces a two-tiered health system, and evokes a bifocal approach to providing treatment. As a consequence, there will be two standards of medical care, with the lower standard afforded to the targeted group whose services are prioritised.[7] The plan needs to be viewed in the light of increasing pressures placed upon physicians to be more cost-effective, and thereby less clinically autonomous.[18] These pressures exist particularly in hospitals and health care centres; there the strain of diminishing budgets has become more visible. For example, critics of Diagnostic Related Groups (DRGs) (a prospective payment plan for Medicare recipients based upon the calculated length of stay and amount of costs in a defined package of hospital services) argue that they place unjustifiable cost-conscious pressures upon physicians which jeopardise the traditional fiduciary relationship between physician and patient. At the same time there is the growing commercialisation of American health care, a result of its strong, free market orientation. The rise of for-profit nursing homes and hospitals attests to American medicine's conversion to a business ethos.

Another fear is that prioritisation will actually work to increase costs. Increased access leads to a greater sum of services.[14] Increased costs can also be the aftermath of pressures exerted from various professional groups to ensure that their services are above the cut-off line. If this is the case, how can there be fair budgeting? SB 27 will extend eligibility from 58% to 100% of the federal poverty level. Yet, the state must still work within a constrained Medicaid budget. There are also pressures from providers, including various specialties such as osteopaths, pharmacists and chiropractors, all vying for their fair share, to maintain adequate reimbursements.[2] Consequently, how can there be a just quality package of basic health care? Taken together, these criticisms lead many to conclude that, in effect, Oregon's plan sustains the existing system. If so, then the plan is counter-productive and works against the implementation of a universal health system.

Responses to the DHHS

There have been some thoughtful responses to the DHHS's August 1992 rejection of Oregon's waiver request. The grounds for rejection indicated the potential for violating ADA tenets, citing the telephone survey's quality of life measurements and the HSC's final 'hand adjustments'. Was the complaint justified?

Capron firmly censures the DHHS allegation. He argues that the use of quality of life gauges does not in itself imply discrimination. There are weaknesses in the administration's stance. First, in its review of the plan, the Office of Technology Assessment's analysis showed that the telephone survey weights had only a minor impact upon the final listing. The HSC itself was criticised for over-using its prerogative at making final adjustments. Next, Capron claims that the DHHS memorandum misconstrues the quality of life measurement. He agreed with Hadorn that the measurement was of 'change in quality of life . . . not the point-in-time quality of life of a patient'. In this respect, it is not discriminatory since it measures the change in health status due to specific treatments, and not the condition itself. Capron adds that, if co-morbidity factors were taken into consideration (and the process was criticised for not doing so), then perhaps the DHHS's claim would have some grounds. Capron's thoughtful analysis raises concerns about the implications of the rejection's rationale. Accordingly, not only has the DHHS 'misrepresented' the spirit of the Oregon plan, but may become a 'virtual road-block' to any rationing strategy.[8]

In Paul Menzel's estimation, even though the DHHS may have misconstrued aspects of the plan, the memorandum raises some tenable issues. Quality of life measurements within a rationing framework pose real dangers. There is a fundamental epistemological difficulty pertaining to knowledge, experience and the sharing of perceptions. Evaluating a condition which one has not experienced is inherently problematic. How do we rank the QWB of others? Menzel stresses the importance of establishing a reasonable conceptual starting point, purged of unnecessary bias. He advises that this starting point encompass not only how we view our current states, but the possibility that we may at some time experience that same state being measured. This problem is compounded when ascertaining the quality of life for early onset congenital conditions. In these cases, evaluators 'would not be making their rationing choices in a fair, risk-taking state of ignorance about how the resulting allocations will turn out individually for them in particular'.[3] In order to judge more properly a condition which we have not experienced, we need to appreciate that experience in a way which balances sufficient knowledge of the condition along with the ability to evaluate reasonably both the effects of that condition and the impact of our judgement upon others.

Furthermore, with respect to the HSC's final 'hand adjustments', using a 'reasonableness' standard according to the six principles mentioned earlier, Menzel is uncomfortable with the incidence principle. Why should periodicity be a relevant factor in prioritisation, especially if the low-incidence condition is inexpensive? Menzel points out that the report may contain a 'subtle bias' in favour of more common conditions, as well as a similar prejudice in favour of communal preferences over individual.

Both Menzel and Capron argue that the examples cited by the DHHS, item 690's liver transplants for alcoholic cirrhosis patients, and item 708's life support for extremely low birth weight babies (under 500 grams), could be fairly resolved. For instance, the plan could distinguish between those with a past alcoholic condition and those with an unrehabilitated condition. In any case, the examples are not blatant illustrations of discrimination.[3,8] In fact, the October 1992 revision does end up funding these two examples by re-ranking them respectively as item 132 (cirrhosis of liver or biliary tract/liver transplant) and item 40 (low birth weight, under 2500 grams/medical therapy).[6]

To conclude, other issues now need to be addressed compelled by the DHHS waiver rejection and the HSC's most recently revised listing. As we stated, the revision encompassed a simplification of the earlier more intricate methodology, the deletion of numeric weights and quality of life descriptors, and line item changes. The HSC believes that despite these modifications, it has remained essentially faithful to its fundamental principles and community values. Yet given the nature of the changes, this remains to be determined. Does the revision demonstrate a virtuous flexibility on the part of the HSC? Or does it portray a capitulation to political pressures which, in effect, compromise its fundamental premises? Are there now two separate prioritisation plans: the original May 1991 initiative along with its October 1992 metamorphosis?

In any case, the overriding merit of the project remains the same: it forces us to confront the agonising dilemma surrounding the rationing of health services. Daniel Callahan notes that any resolution to this dilemma depends upon how we address two fundamental issues. First, is it justifiable to use an imperfect system, such as Oregon's? Next, is it an unacceptable compromise to work within current political and social realities? Callahan feels that what is at issue is not a resulting two-tiered system, but whether the standard package of benefits provided for all will be a decent quality of care. The inability to receive the same kind of health care as the more affluent does not in itself constitute an injustice. 'If the private sector has not learned how to set limits, must the public sector do likewise?'[11] Why should the private sector establish the norm for defining what constitutes basic health care?

This needs to be taken at least one step further. Oregon's strategy tackles a monumental challenge: how is it possible to expand access to quality health care and still manage to control health care spending? Yet, it struggles within the same political and economic environment from which features of the American health care crisis emanate. It ranks treatments according to their overall medical effectiveness, and draws a cut-off line essentially determined by fiscal realities within a market-oriented health system. A pernicious consequence of a market-driven health care system is that it turns out to be ultimately profit-conscious, with services evaluated primarily in terms of their investment return, rather than on health care needs. And problems spiral since we tend to confuse 'health care needs' with 'health-related desires'.[12] Rationing cannot replace the circumstances which give rise to the need for rationing.

Oregon's experiment forces us to face squarely inequities within the current system. Its unique response to its finite budget is not to cut eligibility, or to diminish reimbursements, but to reduce spending for treatments which are considered to be of lowest priority, while access is guaranteed for all. It is a plan worth examining, and deserves the opportunity to stand the test of time and error.

Note

This work was essentially written before the final approval in March 1993. Events from that time on are described in general in the section *Plan Finally Approved*. Therefore, this chapter now covers events up to April 1994.

Acknowledgements

The author thanks Dr Angela Schneider-O'Connell (Bioethics Consultation Group) and Paige Sipes-Metzler (Executive Director, Oregon Health Services Commission) for their helpful guidance, along with the editor and the original reviewers for their valuable comments and assistance.

References

1. Oregon Health Services Commission (1991). *Prioritization of Health Services: A Report to the Governor and Legislature*. Oregon Health Commission, Portland, Oregon.

2. Fox, D.M. and Leichter, H.M. (1991). Rationing care in Oregon: the new accountability. *Health Affairs* **10**(2), 7–27.
3. Menzel, P.T. (1991). Oregon's denial: disabilities and quality of life. *Hastings Center Report* **22**(6), 21–25.
4. Crawshaw, R., Garland, M.J., Hines, B. and Lobitz, C. (1985). Oregon health decisions: an experiment with informed community consent. *Journal of the American Medical Association* **254**(22), 3213–3216. Oregon Health Commission, Portland, Oregon.
5. Hadorn, D.C. (1991). The Oregon priority-setting exercise: quality of life and public policy. *Hastings Center Report* **21**(3), 11–16.
6. Oregon Health Services Commission (1992). *The Oregon Health Plan: Revised Priority List*, 30 October 1992. Oregon Health Commission, Portland, Oregon.
7. Dougherty, C.J. (1991). Setting health care priorities: Oregon's next step. *Hastings Center Report* **21**(3), 1–10.
8. Capron, A.M. (1992). Oregon's disability: principles or politics? *Hastings Center Report* **22**(6), 18–20.
9. Veatch, R.M. (1991). Should basic care get priority? Doubts about rationing the Oregon way. *Kennedy Institute of Ethics Journal* **1**(3), 187–206.
10. Goldsmith, M.F. (1989). Oregon pioneers 'more ethical' Medicaid coverage with priority-setting project. *Journal of the American Medical Association* **262**(2), 176–177.
11. Callahan, D. (1991). Ethics and priority setting in Oregon. *Health Affairs* **10**(2), 78–87.
12. Dougherty, C. J. (1988). *American Health Care: Realities, Rights, and Reforms*, Oxford University Press, New York.
13. Packwood, B. (1990). Oregon's bold idea. *Academic Medicine* **65**(11), 623–633.
14. Brown, L.D. (1991). The national politics of Oregon's rationing plan. *Health Affairs* **10**(2), 28–51.
15. Gore, Jr. A. (1990). Oregon's bold mistake. *Academic Medicine* **65**(11), 634–635.
16. LaPuma, J. and Lawlor, E.F. (1990). Quality adjusted life years: ethical implications for physicians and policymakers. *Journal of the American Medical Association* **263**(21), 2917–2921.
17. Klein, R. (1992). Warning signals from Oregon. *British Medical Journal* **304**, 1457–1458.
18. Nelson, R.M. and Drought, T. (1992). Justice and the moral acceptability of rationing medical care: the Oregon experiment. *Journal of Medicine and Philosophy* **17**(1), 97–117.

Chapter 3

Health Care Reform in the United States: Clinton or Canada?

Lawrence D. Brown and Theodore R. Marmor[*]

School of Public Health, Columbia University, New York, USA
[*]School of Management, Yale University, USA

Part One

THE CLINTON REFORM PLAN'S ADMINISTRATIVE STRUCTURE: THE REACH AND THE GRASP

Lawrence D. Brown and Theodore R. Marmor

Few Americans dispute that their medical care system requires substantial reform. Although the language of crisis is undoubtedly over-used in American politics, there is now a widely shared conviction that medical costs are too high compared to the benefits received, that too many citizens have no (or inadequate) health insurance, and that the complexity of America's financing and reimbursement arrangements bedevils patients, payers and providers to an insufferable degree.

The recent debate about public remedies for these problems, however, satisfied almost no one. Labels and symbols of proposals, not realistic standards for their assessment, dominated the discussion. Indeed, simply getting clear what the President proposed was a major analytical task.

Reforming Health Care: The Philosophy and Practice of International Health Reform.
Edited by D. Seedhouse. © 1995 John Wiley & Sons Ltd.

The Clinton Proposal, and its Theoretical Difficulties

Universal health insurance was America's most critical domestic issue, and as a presidential candidate, Clinton made its passage a top priority. But unhappily, from what we knew of the 'mangaged competition' proposals that emerged from the task force led by Hillary Rodham Clinton and Ira Magaziner, we—even as ardent proponents of universal health insurance—found ourselves hoping for a bit more congressional gridlock. We would still argue for passing the Clinton proposal rather than nothing. But the President's proposal was flawed in ways that have everything to do with means and nothing to do with the basic principles—which are universal insurance and health care of high quality at affordable cost.

Although the President's plan had many good features, it was hardly the brilliant start that reformers anticipated. First, maintaining work-based health insurance would have created unnecessary and costly complexity and depressed the demand for workers. Simplicity should have been one of the highest priorities for reforming a medical care system that spent three times as much on administration as the next worst of the advanced nations. Furthermore, continued financing of health insurance through what amounted to a tax on employment (whether you call it employer mandates or payroll contributions) would have increased unemployment. To be fair, the President knew this. But he stuck with employment-based financing because he feared even more what his political opponents would have done if he proposed a straightforward tax.

The proposals also aimed to reduce costs by changing the behaviour of doctors, hospitals and patients, rather than addressing the complexity of insurance companies and the role of large employers as insurance providers. But this was backward. Such a plan favoured choice of insurance plans but failed to give patients choice precisely where they wanted it—at the point of service. Again, this increased administrative costs while confusing consumers.

The attempt to force patients and physicians into Health Maintenance Organisation (HMO) style practice, including some serious effort to 'manage' the care that is provided, would have interfered with professional judgement and physician–patient autonomy. Once again there was no reason to take this approach. There were plenty of other effective ways to promote preventive medicine and constrain spending. Finally, the Clinton proposals sought to control costs by methods that were known not to work, were uncertain to work or might have severely restricted access to needed care. Managed competition alone clearly does not work, because providers can shift costs. Managed competition combined with an overall restriction on total payments (the apparent Clinton plan) was unproven as a universal system anywhere in the world.

The fallback position of the Clinton plan seemed to be this: constrain costs by restricting the number of procedures, ailments or conditions that universal health insurance will cover. This meant that certain groups would be well served, others less so. And consequently the plan retreated from the promise of universality and required an enormously complex administrative system to set and keep the boundaries between insured and uninsured care. Moreover, this being America, there was certain to be massive litigation about coverage.

The Clinton plan was not just flawed policy, it was also bad politics. It was simply too complex to explain. From the very beginning, the task force refused to consider straightforward, government-administered universal health insurance, saying it was not politically feasible. Instead, they produced a slogan ('managed competition'), inexplicable proposals and a fragile, complicated administrative design.[1]

The Clinton Proposal: Is it Even Workable?

So much for the theory, which received intense coverage in America. Despite this attention, one fundamental set of issues was consistently neglected. How, and how well, would alternative policy options actually be implemented if they were to be adopted?

The focus of the first part of this chapter will be on implementation issues raised by the President's proposal, a matter as crucial to wise policy choice as to improved administration. After all, it would hardly be sensible to assume that one reform plan is superior to another merely because it falls into one category or another. The particulars of a plan—the chances it would prove workable—ought to weigh heavily in evaluating it. In short, we need to move beyond preconceptions of plans to realistic forecasts of their likely implementation.

There is an old public administration saying that public authority must centralise appropriately before it can decentralise effectively. The American polity always has difficulty grasping this truth, and it lies at the heart of the policy challenge to the Clinton reform plan. The problems of American medicine arise substantially from its fragmented, *laissez-faire* character. The main actors (businesses, insurers, providers, governments) play by 'rules' they set by and for themselves with little accountability to the larger public interest (a term so out-of-fashion in the health debate that it has become positively quaint).

The basic challenge to reform is to end *laissez-faire*, which means at long last adopting a firm, coherent framework of federal policy. In our view, that framework must do five things if it is to stand a chance of really repairing America's system of medical care finance and provision. It must:

1. Create a clear universal entitlement to health insurance for all citizens.
2. Define a basic benefits package as to the substance of that entitlement.
3. Establish financing arrangements that put some of society's money where its mouth is.
4. Radically reform present cost-containment mechanisms so that we get affordable universal coverage.
5. Fundamentally simplify the complex world of health insurance.

To its credit, the Clinton plan addressed all five criteria intelligently and in depth, though one could certainly argue with specific details. And for that, *bravo*. But whether the means prescribed to these ends were in fact workable is another matter. What troubled us most about the Clinton proposal was the complex and fragile administrative architecture it erected. The plan bore the marks of its parentage all too plainly: a section for every task force sub-group, the wish lists and speculations of every contributing cadre dutifully displayed with too little regard for what tasks government (federal and state) is likely to perform well and what lies beyond its ken and capacity.

Consider just two illustrations here. The first is risk adjustment, which most experts believe is in a very primitive methodological state. Yet it is crucial to the quality of the 'managed competition' the alliances were to encourage among health insurance plans. Risk adjustment influences the fairness of a plan's remimbursement, its willingness to enrol and serve the disadvantaged, and its financial stability over time. If the methods of risk adjustment are really as shaky as many credible commentators believe, this precondition for the structured shopping for and buying of health insurance was not ready for national prime time.

A second case in point is the monitoring and assurance of quality, the provision of consumer information, and so on. Improving the quality of American medical care is obviously desirable. But our understanding of the rather slow start and modest early returns of the federal practice guidelines and support of outcomes research prompts caution here. The results—in addition to the sectarian sniping between advocates of these respective reform schools—suggested that these capacities should be allowed to mature quietly and gradually on the sidelines of federal policy rather than be hauled onto centre stage for the extensive short-term development and deployment envisioned in the plan. Moreover, the Clinton proposal blurred two distinct issues: the generation of sound scientific data and interpretations to allow experts to assess medical care quality is one thing; working these data and assessments into a form that will be useful to consumer-citizens exercising their options in the medical marketplace is quite another. The point is simple: since wish lists were compiled, the plan's defenders and critics should have distinguished those tasks that the federal and state governments are capable of doing well—or at least adequately—from those that could bedevil and discredit reform. Administrative capacity should have received more sustained attention on its own.

The need for this is clear as soon as one appreciates the extraordinarily speculative administrative infrastructure that held together the various parts of the Clinton proposal. Health policy analysts all too often assume that where there is a strategic will there must be an institutional way, that administrative form readily follows economic function. This faith—which one might regard as the institution equivalent of immaculate conception—generates costly mistakes. The plan's heroic assumptions about institution-building might have worked out well—or they might have produced adminstrative nightmares that undercut the assurances of the security the plan sought to provide. Ordinary Americans surely do not treasure their current encounters with insurers, employers, and providers when trying to piece together coverage and care. But our fear was that as critics depicted the Brave New World citizens would face in the reorganised Clintonian system, we would have heard a lot about the questionable wisdom of living with familiar evils instead of rushing to others we could have hardly imagined. The options for citizens (the menu of plans, prices, plan features, etc.) would have been a result of decisions made on at least four institutional levels. Two of these—the National Health Board and the Health Alliances—would have been brand new and the two others—states and health plans—would have shouldered new and unfamiliar tasks in an unsettled environment.

Care comes first, and most immediately, from the proposed health plan. Despite premature celebration of the managed care 'revolution', most 'plans' are now rather casual and loosely-managed affairs, and few of their managers, let alone subscribers, view them as powerful efficiency-forcing vehicles. These insurance plans (which are themselves exotic in many parts of the country) would have been told to generate low bids and stay within the caps on premium increases that Clinton's schedule of cost deceleration demanded. The ensuing organisational adaptations—which could have hardly avoided sizeable micromanagement of provider and patient behaviour—would have been quite a shock. And those who contended they would prove acceptable because they derive from market forces, not 'obvious' government choices, would have been in for a surprise.

Financial Security or the Ideal System?

Both here and elsewhere health reform debates have a predictable shape. They pit those who believe reform should concentrate on financial security against those who also want to devise an ideal overall system (optimal arrangements of plans, providers, incentives and facilities). The Clinton proposal fell unabashedly in the latter camp. But health reform reached the top of the nation's public agenda not because of dissatisfaction with the structure and organisation of American medicine. The explanation, as Theda Skocpol notes, is that the 'uneasily insured' got upset over the costs and dependability of coverage within a system many of whose features they rather like. If these middle-class Americans interpreted the plan to mean 'You should now have the right to pay through the nose for not joining a group or staff model HMO', the Clinton reform, we believe, would have foundered. But without such pressures ('those who want a more costly plan will pay more' in the gentle lingo of the plan) the cost-containment targets may well be unreachable—at least by market forces.

The health insurance plans themselves were but the tip of the organisational iceberg, however. How the consumer's choice among plans would have worked out depended critically on decisions made by the so-called health alliances. These were inventions made from flimsy theoretical cloth, and remind one uncomfortably of the Health Systems Agencies of the 1970s. Non-profit corporations run by boards of consumers and purchasers would have been a particularly hot political potato. Aside from the difficulty and artificiality of excluding representatives with a tincture of provider affiliation in a society that spends one dollar in seven on medical care, 'consumers' and 'purchasers' are not homogeneous categories. In all such settings, one can expect agitated combat among sub-groups within these camps for 'fair' representation. Nor is it clear how alliances can be held accountable, to whom, and for what. Suppose one does not like an alliance or what it is doing? To whom does one complain? We imagine states managing these conflicts; that suggests making alliance agencies of state government or of the state executive branch. That would presumably enhance accountability and co-ordination with the rest of state health administration. Finally, governance aside, alliances face a long list of complex tasks. These tasks require large and expert staffs, are inherently controversial, and involve the flow of billions of dollars and the medical care of millions of people. How likely are the alliances to know what they are doing and to do it fairly and well given the multiple, conflicting goals—good access, high quality, lower costs, etc.—that comprise their mission? Where will they find the administrative expertise? Is this a sensible way of economising on expertise?

In the Clinton proposal, sitting alongside the plans, alliances, and states like a colossus was a fourth institutional layer—the proposed National Health Board (NHB). This was yet another jerry-built construct handed broad powers and many difficult jobs. It was to oversee the states, interpret, update, and adjust the benefit package, issue regulations for the national budget or its premium cap surrogate and enforce them, set baseline budgets for the alliance, tackle issues of drug pricing, and more. Would the federal government have been able to assemble the administrative talent to do all this well on a national scale within the next few years? The Prospective Payment Commission for hospitals (PROPAC) and the Physician Payment Review Commission (PPRC) are useful but limited precedents; they deal with relatively delimited issues affecting one federal programme insuring America's elderly, Medicare. The NHB would have been obliged among many other things to promulgate risk adjustment methods for a national system of alliances, leaving the states to use these methods or seek a waiver to substitute their own. States and alliances would have faced intense pressures over the choices of methods with different distributional consequences, and one could picture federal/state battles over waivers. Multiplying these potential inter-governmental conflicts by the rest of the NHB's tasks leaves you with administrative chaos. Also troubling was the structural fragmentation the system retained in the aggregate: oversight of regional alliances by the NHB, corporate alliances by the Department of Labour, Medicare with the Department of Health and Human Services (DHHS), and so on. Who would fit these pieces together? Would it matter much? Critics charged that the promised administrative simplification ironically entailed stacking upon untested public and quasi-public enterprises that, in the aggregate, create a merely formal security.

Aside from the many strengths of the Clinton plan, the downside is that it appeared to reflect a limited and constrained policy analysis that concentrated too much on preferred strategic options, the 'what' issue of public choice. It paid too little realistic attention to 'who' and 'how' questions and to the light these cast on the feasibility of initial policy choices. Whether and to what degree one can accomplish a task has everything to do with calculations of its desirability. The structural and implementation questions—addressing matters that can shape outcomes decisively—must focus on the limits of administrative capacity, on the workability of organisational missions and the technologies that advance them, and on the complexities of the operational challenges that descend on the federal system and the public and private sectors.

'Analytical' policy reasoning—identifying a wide range of strategic options and reviewing the costs and benefits of each—is not so much faulty as fundamentally incomplete. Wise policy choice involves pondering problems and programmes through several conceptual lenses, among which administrative and organisational perspectives should be prominent. It would have been sad if the Clinton health reforms had had an aftermath like that of many of America's great society programmes. In the late 1960s and early 1970s legions of implementation scholars ventured forth, with neo-conservatives close behind, to document in depressingly vivid detail that the federal government was throwing at many problems money that state, local, and private sector implementors squandered for want of reachable goals, manageable tasks, and coherent administrative structures. Such risks were all over the Clinton reform plan and alarmed those who shared fully its admirable aims. Equally important, the plan's institutional complexity—whatever its origins in calculations that less fragile administrative designs were politically infeasible—fundamentally impaired the mobilisation of citizen consent to health reform itself.

On this view, administrative simplification should have been a central object of congressional adjustment. Revisions should have kept clearly in mind the five crucial reform aims noted earlier: universal coverage, a basic benefits package, a sound financing framework, radical insurance reform, and cost-containment with teeth. One could insist upon these five principles (however further explicated) and, Canada-like, gamble that relatively unfettered federalism can work. This meant that states, as they saw fit, would have had to figure out how to design systems meeting the five 'principles'.

Or, the federal framework could offer three broad options: for example, a single-payer plan, an alliance-based form of managed competition, or all-payer rate setting. This, of course, means that the Clinton 'solution' would become an option, not a requirement for the 50 states without a special waiver. The prospect of some 200 non-profit corporations handling billions of dollars of health funds and wielding enormous market clout, is in many respects terrifying. The difficulty of monitoring 50 distinct systems would probably not be greater than that of assessing and enforcing the compliance of 50 systems with a detailed federal blueprint. And broader flexibility reduces risks that were very real in the Clinton plan: namely, endless new battles over federal waivers for state variations, a source of conflict that has sorely oppressed the states in recent years.

It goes without saying that the Clinton administration's plan (and planning) forced medical care reform onto the nation's public agenda, which was exactly where it should have been. And it also should be said that much of the carping about the costs or complexity of the Clinton plan was transparently disingenuous, comparing it to another nirvana and ignoring the brutal realities of contemporary costs and current complexity. But administrative chaos was not a price worth paying at one of the few political moments when substantial change seemed possible. What the Congress and administration should have done, and still should do, is reshape the administration's design of the Clinton plans while holding firm to its goals.

Part Two

PATTERNS OF FACT AND FICTION IN THE USE OF CANADIAN EXPERIENCE

Theodore R. Marmor

In the summer of 1994, the US preoccupation with health care reform hardly seemed to involve Canada. During the campaign of 1992 candidate Clinton repeatedly cited the superior experience of other industrial democracies in controlling health costs, including Canada's Medicare. But he seldom embraced Medicare as a model of national health insurance. Indeed, one noticed his innocent repetition of some of the myths which the American Medical Association (AMA) and the Health Insurance Association of America (HIAA) have, along with others, relentlessly disseminated during the most recent period of political interest in Canada, which roughly extended from 1989 to early 1992. But Canada has played a crucial if not well-understood role in American debates over health care since the late 1960s and, even today, has an influence that is all too easy to overlook.

The history of US interest in Canadian public health insurance is mostly a story of episodes of public discussion and interest (1970–74; 1989–92) punctuated by longer periods of inattention. Before the 1970s, very few health policy analysts in the US knew much about the Canadian experience or paid much attention to it. Among the exceptions were scholars like Cecil Sheps and Sam Wolfe, Canadians who participated in Canada's reforms during the post-war period, emigrated to the US, and continued to write about the Canadian experience and its relevance to the US. But the number was small.

But that was not to remain true in the 1970s. Early in the decade, Senator Ted Kennedy was but the most prominent example of the many politicians who travelled north to marvel at Canada's relative success and celebrated its lessons upon return. In 1973 and 1974, national health insurance was firmly on the American political agenda, and the Kennedy–Corman plan of that period owed much to the Canadian model. The 1975 book *Canadian National Health Insurance: Lessons for the United States* was widely read in academic and policy circles, and Canadian scholars like Bob Evans of the University of British Columbia were regular participants in seminars and conferences south of their border.[2]

Yet, it took until 1989 for a serious interest in Canadian Medicare to reappear. And, then, it emerged in a familiar manic-depressive cycle of initial excitement, manic coverage, and depressive reaction. The precipitants of excitement are easy enough to identify. In 1989, Lee Iacocca, the head of Chrysler, and his board member and former Carter cabinet officer, Joseph Califano, published admiring editorials in the *New York Times*. Though nothing new was being said, new figures were arguing that Canada's form of national health insurance combined broader coverage and less cost than in the US and, furthermore, that our persistent medical inflation was a serious problem for the competitiveness of US corporations. What then followed was a torrent of attention—from squads of congress people visiting Montreal, Toronto, and Vancouver to numerous newspaper features, from the Public Broadcasting System's 1990 documentary *Borderline Medicine* to the persistently favourable reviews of Canadian experience by a new medical group, Physicians for a National Health Plan (PNHP). All three television networks did specials on Canada's experience with Medicare, and for a time, Canadian experts were inundated with requests for interviews, information, and expertise. Had the 1992 election been held in 1990, Canada would have figured prominently in it.

The forces of reaction, however, had ample time to develop. Led by the AMA initially, the critics of Canada's 'socialised medicine' used the full arsenal of propagandistic techniques to question both Canada's performance and its relevance to the US.* The HIAA came to take the lead role here, shamelessly blasting a favourable report by the Government Accounting Office in 1991 as 'partisan'. A pattern emerged: any news story in Canada about waiting lists, a disappointed patient or physician, or squabbles about the availability of funds for doctors, hospitals, or capital quickly found its place in the testimony of the HIAA, the American Farm Bureau Federation, and right-wing think-tanks like the Heritage Foundation. Naive journalists, using the shopworn technique of quoting 'both sides', gave ample space to both the celebrators and the detractors, thereby repeating myths without analysing them. The public paid less attention to this than the politicians, overwhelmingly stating their approval of the Canadian programme pollsters described to them. But the growth of a vigorous pro- and anti-Canada lobby took its toll on risk-averse presidential candidates.

All of this was played out in dramatic form during the Democratic primaries of 1992. Senator Kerry, an admirer of Canadian health insurance, advanced a plan similar to Medicare, but increasingly distanced himself from explicit citation of the model. He came to talk, as did others, of the need for an 'American solution' for an 'American problem', hoping to avoid the knee-jerk nativism that rises close to the surface of American public life whenever it is claimed that another nation has something to teach it. And with that came additional commentary that Canada, after all, was really quite different from the US. Seymour Martin Lipset, a thoughtful and nuanced commentator on North American similarities and differences, had recently published his *Continental Divide*,[3] which carefully and sensibly addressed the differences across the borders. But the advocates of market solutions to medical problems seized on this and other Canadian materials to argue that, however good Canada's Medicare might be, it was the product of a nation committed to 'peace, order and good government', not the US individualistic creed of 'life, liberty, and the pursuit of happiness'.

By December 1992, the vice-president of the HIAA complacently stated on Cable News Network that the 'American people are not ready for a Canadian-

---

* In fairness, the AMA retreated from its propaganda attacks in 1989 after receiving serious criticism from both Canadian physicians and American groups. By 1992, the AMA was taking a far more considered position on universal health insurance, leaving the HIAA as the leading pressure group critical of Canadian Medicare.

style government solution'. And, as the *New York Times* celebrated 'managed competition', their editorial writer persistently dismissed the 'bureaucratic' solution of Canada. Voices of reason persisted, but the undeniable fact is that Canada's Medicare was not a leading contender for the reform soul of President Clinton.

Does this mean that the Canadian experience was rendered useless or its impact reduced to the musings of scholars? I think not, but explaining how is not simple. But consider that, in 1991, journalists assumed that 'play or pay' plans were likely to emerge from the play of American politics, and none of them even mentioned the category of a 'global budget'. In 1994, most journalists were commenting on the possibility of 'managed competition within the context of a global budget', repeating the very words President Clinton used in the last weeks of his campaign. The principles announced by the presidential transition team on health included universality, global budget limits, state involvement, comprehensive benefits, and managed care. All but the last reflect Canadian principles! And the pairing of global budgets and universality reflects the seeping into the US reform mind of precisely the key elements analysts of Canadian experience have been emphasising for two decades. It is true that the decreased appeal (to politicians) of the single-payer model has discouraged many citizen activist groups who know the American public is well disposed to Canada's experience and anxious to rid it of the wasteful administrative expense of 1500 private insurers. But it would be a great mistake to overlook the impact that Canadian experience has had or believe that the labels used to refer to a reform plan fully illuminate its features or the forces that produced them.

Can the United States Learn from Abroad?

Canada, France, and Germany provide their citizens with universal health insurance coverage at a cost of between 8 and 9.5% of gross national product (GNP). Britain, Japan, and Australia provide it for between 6 and 8% of GNP. The US, as is so often noted, spends more than 14% of GNP on health care—more than any other country—and yet ranks below all members of the Organisation for European Co-operation and Development in terms of infant mortality and life expectancy. Yet for all the money spent, there are still some 35 million Americans without health insurance and an undetermined number who have inadequate insurance. The US is obviously doing something wrong.

When other countries achieve what the US says it would like to attain, it makes good sense to look abroad. But for Americans there are particularly revealing difficulties in looking abroad for lessons—whether in government or commerce. The American public is somewhat skittish about America's uniqueness, educated to believe in a special mission and character of this 'city on a hill'. Cross-national comparisons can easily arouse xenophobia, with defenders of the status quo ever ready to invoke the claim that 'America is just different'.

Those of us who do look abroad see three questions as we examine the Canadian health care experience. The first is whether Canada's medical care system is truly exemplary and worth importing. The second is whether a Canadian-style programme is politically feasible in the US. And third, even if desirable as a model and politically acceptable, can Canadian national health insurance be adapted to American circumstances?

Canada's Exemplary Performance

The basic outline of Canada's national health insurance is clear. The federal government conditionally promises each province that it will prepay roughly 40% of the costs of all necessary medical care. The federal grant is available so long as the province's health insurance programme is universal (covering all citizens), comprehensive (covering all conventional hospital and medical care), accessible (no limits on services and no extra charges to patients), portable (each province recognises the others' coverage), and publicly administered (under control of a public, non-profit organisation). All 10 provinces maintain health insurance plans satisfying these criteria. The provincial ministry of health is the only payer in each province. There are no complex eligibility tests or complicated definitions of insured services. Administrative costs, as a consequence, are negligible by American standards.

The practical dynamics of Canada's programme are also simple, at least in outline. Annual negotiations between provincial governments and the providers of care determine hospital budgets and the level of physicians' fees. As in the US, most hospitals are non-profit community institutions and physicians practise (under fee-for-service payment) in diverse individual and group settings. Patients choose their own doctors; doctors bill the province; and hospitals work from global budgets, not itemised billings. Disagreements over insurance claims, gaps in coverage, and bureaucratic incomprehensibility are, for practical purposes, non-existent. Canadian patients and providers never have to file multiple claims to different insurers. (American Medicare beneficiaries might well have to file claims with three or more insurers, and a physician or hospital treating Medicaid patients might have to wait six months or more for payment.)

Most of the negative effects economic theory and Canadian doctors predicted—worrisome physician flight, rationing of life-saving care, long queues, and technological obsolescence—have not emerged. There is, and has always been, some movement of highly trained, highly prized personnel from Canada to the US, and physicians are no exception. But this trend was not greatly affected by Canadian national health insurance, and the numbers have always been small, not enough to offset a steady increase in the number of practising physicians. As Table 1 shows, Canada's physician population ratio has been, and remains, comparable to that of the US.

At the outset, the existing physician fee schedules of provincial medical associations were accepted by the provincial governments, although in most provinces payments were initially set somewhat below 100% to reflect the elimination of a doctor's risk of unpaid debts. Since that time, changes in the fee schedules have been negotiated by provincial medical associations and ministries

Table 1   Physicians per 100 000 people, US and Canada

Year	US	Canada
1965	155	130
1970	159	146
1975	178	172
1980	201	184
1985	224	206
1987	234	216

Data from Organisation for Economic Co-operation and Development (1990). From *Health Care Systems in Transition: The Search for Efficiency*. Paris, OECD, Tables 27 and 61.

of health. The typical process of setting fees is one of extended negotiation, not unilateral imposition. Physicians were the highest paid professionals in Canada before the introduction of universal medical insurance; they still are.

Rationing Care

Canada does ration medical care. So does the US and every other country in the world. What counts is not the presence of rationing (or allocation) but the basis for and the extent of restricted access to health care. The US continues to ration by the ability to pay—a process largely determined by race, class, and employment circumstances. Access to care and the quality of care vary enormously, and many in the US—particularly the poor or poorly insured—experience long waiting lists and substandard facilities, if they receive care at all. By contrast, Canada and most other developed countries try to provide a more uniform standard of care to the entire population. Medical care is allocated largely on the basis of relative medical need, which is determined by physician judgement, not by insurance status, bureaucratic rules, or arbitrary age limits.

At certain times and in some places, substantial waiting lists for selected surgical and diagnostic procedures occur. But the overall rates of hospital use per capita are considerably higher in Canada than in the US. Most patients are cared for in a timely manner, and long waiting lists reflect managerial problems more than chronic shortages of facilities. Emergency care is available immediately to everyone.

There is no question that some expensive, high-technology items are not as available in Canada as they are in the US. Canada has a full range of high-technology facilities, but in considerably less abundance and with little competition for market share. Expensive capital equipment is first approved

Table 2   Comparative availability of selected medical technologies US and Canada (Units per million people)

Medical Technology	US	Canada	Ratio: US/Canada
Open-heart surgery	3.26	1.23	2.7:1
Cardiac catheterisation	5.06	1.50	3.4:1
Organ transplantation	1.31	1.08	1.2:1
Radiation therapy	3.97	0.54	7.4:1
Extracorporeal shock wave lithoscopy	0.94	0.16*	5.9:1
Magnetic resonance imaging	3.69	0.46	8.0:1

United States data are for 1987, Canada for 1989, except where indicated.
* 1988.
Source: D.A. Rublee (1989). Medical technology in Canada and the US. *Health Affairs*, **Fall**, p. 180, reproduced with permission.

only for highly specialised centres, and subsequent diffusion is closely controlled by provincial ministries of health. This control results in lower rates of use for some technologies in Canada—cardiac surgery, magnetic resonance imaging, lithoscopy, and so on (see Table 2). This is not necessarily a bad thing. Throughout North America, there is concern about the appropriate use of expensive new procedures. Inappropriate use is both financially costly and medically dangerous to patients.

The quality of a nation's health care is never simple to measure. Many critics view the slower diffusion and limited use of some new technologies in Canada as evidence of lower quality care. If quality is defined as more high-technology services regardless of relative effectiveness, then the US certainly offers higher quality medical care. If, however, quality is defined by health results rather than by the use of high technology, then there is no evidence of a Canadian disadvantage. If life expectancy and infant mortality measure the quality of a health care system, Canada has a definite advantage. And if consumer satisfaction is a critical component of quality, then both polls and political behaviour put Canadian national health insurance well in the lead.

The generally high levels of Canadian satisfaction suggest the importance of the way health care quality is distributed. When quality is defined as the best technologies and facilities available to the most privileged members of a population, rather than as the facilities available to the average individual, American medical care ranks among the best in the world. But major aspects of American medical care—the limited extent of immunisation, the large number of pregnant women without regular medical attention, and the risk of bankruptcy from illness—would be considered intolerable in other comparably wealthy countries. Canada has fewer centres of technological excellence, but the average level of care is, by any definition, at least equal to that in the US.

Adapting Canada's Health Care System

What would make the Canadian option not only more attractive to the American electorate, but also easier to implement in the American context? Part of the answer lies in distinguishing the necessary from the incidental elements of the Canadian success story in universal health insurance. The Canadian programme combines three features that have made its cost, access, and quality acceptable over nearly 20 years of full-scale operation.

One of the features is universality of coverage. All Canadians are insured on the 'same terms and conditions'. This universality has made it politically impossible in Canada to deal with cost pressures by stealth or to permit end runs around the controls. Second, there is a clear centre of financial responsibility in Canada: a ministry of health or its equivalent in each province. Financing medical care under concentrated rather than fragmented auspices is crucial to the third component of Canada's system: clear political accountability for the cost and quality of and access to Canadian medical care. These three features—universal access, a responsible financing agency, and accountable political leaders to answer for the balance among cost, quality, and access—explain why Canada's performance has been superior to that of the US.

But what do these features of the Canadian model mean for possible American adaptations? What sort of changes could be made without losing what has been necessary for Canada's relatively successful experience with national health insurance?

Canada's universalism is strong in two ways. Every Canadian is literally on the same provincial health insurance plan as his or her neighbour—the equivalent of every Californian belonging to one Blue Cross/Blue Shield plan. What's more, Canadians have the same coverage under their provincial plan: 'equal terms and conditions', not varied options. In the health sphere, Canada is probably more egalitarian than any other comparable industrial democracy. Private insurers are forbidden by law to sell supplementary coverage for publicly insured services. And to maintain the 'equal terms' of access, Canadian doctors since 1984 have for all practical purposes been prevented from charging patients anything above the government's fee schedule.

Not all of these Canadian features are necessary for an acceptable form of universal health insurance. Canada did not start with such a firmly egalitarian version. The Hall Commission of 1964 to 1966, the royal commission that justified extending government hospital insurance to medical care, defined universal coverage as no less than 95% of the citizens in each province. While desirable on egalitarian grounds, literal universality has not been a necessary feature of Canada's success. American reformers need not insist on Canada's strong contemporary form of universal enrolment.

'Uniform' conditions would also be less compelling than in Canada. For Americans to be in the same boat does not necessarily require that the boat's cabins all be the same size or have the same view. What is essential is that the health insurance boat include most Americans on roughly comparable terms.

It is on the issue of the terms of benefits and the constraints on 'supplementation' that the most acrimonious disputes are likely to break out. Could the US (or a state) forego the Canadian ban on supplementary health insurance for services covered under a universal plan without losing financial control? Would it be unacceptable to permit physicians (or other medical professions paid under fee-for-service arrangements) to charge their patients more than the agreed-on schedule of fees?

The answer here is ambiguous. On the first point, Canada has never experimented. But other nations with acceptable national health insurance programmes have supplementary insurance that coexists with public coverage. As for charges that are above negotiated rates ('extra-billing' or 'balance-billing' in the jargon of health economics), the answer is clearer. The ability to contain medical costs depends on establishing firm limits; extra-billing violates those limits and reintroduces barriers to access that universal health insurance is meant to lower. No successful national health insurance programme has permitted this practice for long; Canada found over time that balance-billing became a serious problem in many communities, threatening both the uniformity of treatment and the access to treatment itself. Both supplementary insurance and extra-billing, when widespread, threaten equitable cost control.

Financing National Health Care

Whether Canada's concentration of finance in provincial ministries of health has been crucial to its successful control of medical care costs is the second issue to evaluate. Is the location of responsibility at the provincial as opposed to federal level vital? The other key question is whether Canada's public financing and direct governmental administration are required for political accountability: an identifiable budget accounts for jurisdiction's overall health expenditure.

The cross-national evidence on the first question suggests that it is the concentration of financial responsibility, not its precise location, that is crucial to countervailing inflationary health care cost pressures. Canada, by constitutional requirement, had no choice but to use provincial governments to administer health insurance. Great Britain, by contrast, concentrates financial responsibility in the national Ministry of Health, and Sweden does so in each of its county councils. The lesson for the US is that there are options.

The second, more difficult question concerns the direct accountability of the processes by which health care funds are raised and spent. Public financing makes Canadian outlays for health highly visible. At the same time, Canadian provinces could, and some did, use pre-existing health insurance companies as political buffers between physicians and the government. In the mid-1960s, Ontario used these intermediaries to manage the flow of funds and the processing claims. Such a buffer seemed important then as a concession to the deep hostility many Canadian doctors felt regarding government medical insurance. In fact, the Canadian provinces that used financial intermediaries at the outset abandoned them after a few years. They made administration complicated and more expensive, and once their role in moderating conflict was no longer necessary, they seemed useless (except to the insurance companies).

One can certainly imagine the use of such intermediaries in the US. This, after all, has been the pattern with American Medicare since 1965—an arrangement that draws on private expertise and 'economises' on the number of public employees. Canadians found such indirect management cumbersome and more expensive to manage than direct administration. But contracting out financial tasks is certainly, on the Canadian evidence, compatible with political accountability.

In the US of the 1990s, however, the crucial political problem facing national health insurance advocates is the public's hostility toward increased taxes. Can one imagine Canadian-style government health insurance working without direct public finance? In other words, what would be lost if, for example, state regulatory authorities set the terms of medical care financing, negotiated with hospitals and physicians, and required that employers finance health insurance directly or pay into a state fund a fixed amount per employee? However the point is phrased, the question remains the same: is it possible to have the right level of countervailing power without the fusion of taxing and negotiating responsibility?

The answer to that question is far from obvious. In some European countries—Germany in particular—national and state governments have played a powerful regulatory role without Canada's single-payer feature. The German government constrains the negotiations among physicians, hospitals, and the thousands of sickness funds without channelling social insurance financing through conventional public tax accounts. It sets the rules by which the parties operate, and each of the sickness funds faces the full financial consequences of its members' medical care. There is both financial accountability and complicated administration in the German example. What the US should notice is that it does not have the German history of lifelong involvement with one health insurance institution.

What this suggests is that the degree of responsibility for health financing—and the clarity about where that accountability lies—is not solely determined by the details of public finance. There are forms of mandated health insurance, which finances care on terms negotiated by public officials, that might closely resemble in practice the publicly financed, compulsory health insurance programme found in Canada.

It is certainly possible to imagine mandated universal health insurance—with workable regulations drawn from German experience—working tolerably well in the US. Such arrangements could address the problems of inflation, inadequate coverage, and political accountability, but less effectively than a system modelled after Canada's. The US should be under no illusion here; there are choices available, with different trade-offs among acceptability, effectiveness, and administrative complexity. What the US has at the moment is a vicious circle of trouble; a system like Canada's is possible, but a less direct programme would be an improvement.

This sort of reasoning led some policy analysts to suggest adapting the Canadian model along the lines suggested earlier. Their proposal treats the state health department as the negotiating agent of universal health insurance, insurance made universal by the accretion of mandated coverage for workers and their families, Medicare for those over 65 and the disabled, Medicaid for the poor, and a new insurance plan for those not in these categories. No one starting from a blank slate would seek this rather complicated version of universal coverage through aggregation, clear public responsibility for costs, and decentralised administration. But, as a third choice, it should be tolerable.[4]

The Case of the Canadian Model

In the early 1970s, American experts paid considerable attention to Canada's recently completed programme of national health insurance. That scrutiny was part of the substantial interest in an American form of universal health insurance. When the realities of stagflation in the 1970s and early 1980s removed national health insurance from the American political agenda, the lessons of Canada's experience were put aside, hardly noticed except by specialists in health policy. The reawakening of American interest in Canada comes without anything like a widely shared American appreciation of how Canadian health insurance works in practice.

The result of that disparity between interest and knowledge is a very uneven discussion of what the US can and cannot learn from its neighbour to the north, let alone what adaptations to American circumstances a conscious effort to borrow from Canada's example would entail. Instead, the discussion of Canadian health insurance resembles a shouting match: enthusiasts pointing to evidence about citizen satisfaction and relatively low expenditures per capita, and detractors arguing either that Canada is too different for the US to take seriously as a model or that the model itself is terrible because it creates long waiting lists, causes doctors to emigrate, and disappoints patients.

If there is any country from which the US can learn, it is Canada. Having had similar medical care arrangements for most of the 20th century, Canada and the US have conducted over the past 20 years a fateful experiment in forms of medical finance. It is two decades and hundreds of billions of dollars too late to contend that the US should have acted on Canadian lessons in the early 1970s. That option simply was not politically available in the economic aftermath of the first oil crisis in 1973. But that does not mean, in the 1990s and beyond, that Americans cannot learn from Canada's example.

The central lesson of the Canadian experiment is that the balance among cost, quality, and access is relatively easy to evaluate. What Canada illustrates clearly is that a sensibly organised national health insurance system can work in a political community similar to that in the US, that universal coverage, coherent financial responsibility, and clear political accountability are the central ingredients of success, and that a population accustomed to the same standard of medical care as the US can take pride in what in essence are 10 provincial Blue Cross/Blue Shield plans with comprehensive benefits to which everyone belongs as a matter of right. If that were understood clearly, the problems of adapting the Canadian model to America would seem less daunting.

References and Notes

1. Marmor, T.R. and Mashaw, J.L. (1993). A little gridlock might help. *LA Times*, 15 August.
2. Andreopolus, S. ed. (1975). *Canadian National Health Insurance: Lessons for the United States*, John Wiley and Sons, New York. The sequel to this work, *Medicare at Maturity* (1984), Evans, R.G. and Stoddart, G.L. (eds), University of Calgary Press, Calgary, was far less well known, published as it was during the Reagan years.
3. Lipset, S.M. (1990). *Continental Divide: The Values and Institutions in the United States and Canada*, Routledge, New York.
4. Marmor, T.R. (1991). *The Future of American Medical Care*. Testimony before the Joint Economic Committee of the Congress of the United States, 2 October.

This article, updated and slightly revised, is taken from: Marmor, T.R. (1993). Health care reform in the United States: patterns of fact and fiction in the use of Canadian experience. *American Review of Canadian Studies* 23(1), 47–64. It constitutes Ch. 12 of T.R. Marmor's (1994) book of essays, *Understanding Health Care Reform*, Yale University Press, New Haven.

Chapter 4

Health Care Reform in the UK: Working for Patients?

*David Gladstone and Michael Goldsmith**

Department of Social Policy, University of Bristol, UK
*Sedgwick Noble Lowndes Health Care Ltd., London, UK

Introduction

> The proposals . . . offer new opportunities, and pose new challenges, for everyone
> concerned with the running of the Service.   *Margaret Thatcher*[1]

The years between 1988 and 1990 witnessed a restructuring of the British Welfare State. Health care was part of that process, but it also included school-age education and social services. Whilst the predisposing factors may not have been identical, certain elements of change were common to all sectors.

> In each case state finance . . . was to be retained; but the system of service provision
> was to change often radically . . . the state was to become primarily only a
> purchaser of welfare services, with state provision being systematically replaced
> by a system of independent providers competing with one another in internal or
> quasi markets.[2]

In health care the effect of such changes has been to replace the 40-year-old command-and-control bureaucratic planning system with a planned or quasi-market model designed 'to expose providers to competitive tests of cost-effectiveness and quality while retaining safeguards for the consumer.'[3]

Against that background, the purpose of this chapter is to describe and attempt an evaluation of the recent changes introduced into the British National Health Service (NHS). In doing so, it will concentrate on the debate surrounding health care reform that developed during the 1980s and the changes initiated by the Conservative government in the first part of the NHS and Community Care Act 1990 which came into effect in April 1991. Central to those reforms was the

Reforming Health Care: The Philosophy and Practice of International Health Reform.
Edited by D. Seedhouse. © 1995 John Wiley & Sons Ltd.

creation of an internal market by means of the separation of the purchaser and provider function, the creation of NHS 'trust' hospitals and the introduction of budget-holding general practitioners (GPs).

'Taken together the proposals represent the most far-reaching reform of the National Health Service in its 40-year history.' That was how Prime Minister Margaret Thatcher described the changes in her Foreword to the government's White Paper *Working for Patients* which was published in January 1989. But how far have the essential features of the post-Second World War creation of the NHS altered as a result of these recent changes? It remains a tax-funded service free to the user at the point of demand and much of the commercial rhetoric of the White Paper has become the practice of managed competition, a quasi-market with a continuing role of considerable (some free marketeers would say excessive) importance for central government. If its essential features apparently remain little changed, how far have the NHS reforms altered the culture of professional practice and created a health care system which is more effectively working for patients? These are the elements of the evaluation which will be considered in this chapter.

Background Influences

We have to sweep away myths, dispense with several sacred cows and conduct our discussions rationally . . . outdated ideology must not be allowed to stand in the way.   *John Moore*[4]

Whilst the National Health Service has continually suffered from attempts at its reform since the early 1960s, with successive governments introducing changes aimed at making the service more efficient, or realistically cost-effective, the Thatcher government never really had any intention of carrying out such a reform during its first decade in office.

Thatcher actively disliked the politics of health care and found professional groups like the doctors difficult to deal with. She had no real understanding of the minutiae of health issues except that ever-increasing amounts of money had to be found from the public purse to fund the NHS.

It came as some surprise, therefore, when the issues of the NHS and its funding blew up to crisis level in the winter of 1987 and 1988. This reticence on behalf of the Prime Minister was at variance with the views of many of the 'right wing' think-tanks associated with the Tory party who had been advocating the need for real reforms in the funding and delivery of health care.

Despite NHS reform being on the agenda, and within John Moore's speech at the 1987 Conservative party conference, nevertheless it is clear that the Prime Minister would have proceeded more cautiously to reform had the crisis or, more accurately, the perceived crisis, not become increasingly prominent in the media in the winter months of 1987–8.

There had been increasing problems from the mid-1980s onwards with hospital and ward closures. In December 1982 a national newspaper survey showed that over 3000 hospital beds in England had been closed through lack of money or manpower, and not through lack of need. Shortly after this Tony Newton, Minister of Health, awarded an extra £90 million to the NHS 'to meet the immediate problems'. But it was already clear to the Prime Minister that her continual increases in funding were not actually producing any real benefits in either improved or increased volumes of care. Nor were they achieving the political benefits of stemming the unending criticism of the government's health policies. In the end, it was the storm around the cardiac care, or apparent lack of it, for a child in Birmingham which was the straw that broke the 'health camel's' back.

Advisers to the 10 Downing Street Policy Unit were asked, early in 1988, to recommend urgent political action. It soon became clear that another Royal Commission was unsuitable because of time delays. Whilst the *British Medical Journal* was declaring, in an editorial full of the portents of doom, that the NHS was moving towards terminal decline, the government announced that a confidential review team, chaired by the Prime Minister, would meet regularly in Whitehall and announce its findings later in the year. This decision alone stemmed the tide of criticism and started a barrage of ideas, the like of which had never been seen since the creation of the NHS.

Every think-tank and interested party was to present both to government and the media (usually the latter first) their particular plan for the NHS or, conversely, their reason for preserving the status quo. The Labour party, through their spokesman Frank Dobson, loudly proclaimed that 'it's not broken, do not fix it'. The Labour party's strategy indeed seemed to be one of denying the need for reform but extolling the virtues of providing more central funding for the service. Their view was that the problems were solely financial.

This was certainly not the first time that a perceived or real NHS crisis, whether of funding or management, had led to the institution of a review. In 1953 the Guillebaud Committee was commissioned by Iain Macleod to investigate rises in the cost of the NHS. Harold Wilson instituted the Royal Commission on the NHS in 1975 after what, retrospectively in most eyes, had been a disastrous reorganisation in 1974, largely based on the findings of the American consultant, McKinseys. In that reorganisation the old hospital management boards, which individually managed local hospitals, and the GP local executive councils which ran primary care services, were abolished and replaced by regional, area and district health authorities and family practitioner committees. The area tier of NHS administration was itself abolished by the Conservative government in 1982.

As part of their value-for-money policy, so loudly trumpeted in the early 1980s, the Conservatives introduced many income generation schemes into the NHS. Unfortunately, these never produced the types of revenue savings which ministers had hoped for. At the same time, a policy of contracting out services became increasingly attractive to the government. By 1985 health authorities were required to put out their laundry, cleaning and catering services to competitive tender. This began to pave the way for the main tenet of the 1988 review: the internal market. The notion that the health authorities did not have an inalienable requirement to deliver services themselves but that they were principally in existence to finance and manage the provision of services thus became prevalent. In ways such as these did the seeds of the idea of separating purchasing from providing spring to life.

Throughout 1988 the review team met in the Cabinet Room at 10 Downing Street; but by mid-year no real decisions had been made. John Moore's indecision, and later his illness, resulted in his removal and replacement by Kenneth Clarke, who had gained previous ministerial experience at the Department of Health. Influential papers from the Institute of Economic Affairs, the Adam Smith Institute and the Centre for Policy Studies,[5-9] all advocating the type of internal markets which had originally been suggested by Professor Alain Enthoven in 1985,[10] gained both publicity and ascendancy in the race for ideas. At the same time, the Moore-led idea of switching from tax-based to insurance-based funding as well as an internal market for provision, became less acceptable to the Treasury and hence to the review team.

Finally after many detailed discussions, in the autumn of 1988 the government decided that the ideas of self-governing hospitals and GP fund-holders as a route for the internal market would be the most successful basis for the reforms. In a blaze of publicity in January 1989, the White Paper *Working for Patients* was published amid television roadshows and, for the government, uniquely user-friendly brochures. The new market-led NHS had been re-born.

Proposals and Legislation

The impressive fact remains that the will of the politicians, the thraldom of policy makers and the collaboration of the managers held sufficiently . . . to ensure that legislation was passed and acted upon.   *John Butler*[11]

From an ideological point of view, the market economy in health care was not actually a very radical idea for the Thatcher government. They had already introduced the philosophy and structures of general management into the NHS in the mid-1980s, after the *Griffiths Report* had been published in October 1983. At the same time, the Resource Management Institute (RMI) had been started in six pilot hospitals in 1986. The idea of RMI was to improve the rather inadequate information technology for patient care available in hospitals. In addition, Mrs Thatcher herself had been particularly impressed with the success of the measures which had been taken to divert cash direct to hospitals from the Treasury as part of the waiting list initiative. Mrs Thatcher felt that the circumvention of the bureaucracy of the NHS to get money direct to the providers was very impressive.

It is not surprising, therefore, that the foundation stones of the internal market were to separate the providers from the purchasers. It was felt by the majority of advisers to the review that the principle of central funding by government of the vast majority of NHS care should continue, but health care provision should be carried out by providers in competition with each other in a real market. The White Paper *Working for Patients* was thus a great political success. It allowed government to open the NHS to competitive market forces whilst still continuing the hallowed 'free at the point of use' tax-funded principle.

The main proposals were, in the White Paper's own words, to secure two objectives.

1. To give patients, wherever they live, better health care and greater choice of services available.
2. To produce greater satisfaction and rewards for NHS staff who successfully respond to local needs and preferences.[12]

The White Paper contained several key measures.

1. More delegation of responsibility to local level: responsibilities were delegated from region to district and from district to hospital.
2. Self-governing hospitals were formed. NHS hospital trusts were created by transferring hospital management and ownership to a trust with centrally and locally appointed directors.
3. New funding arrangements were created by making money follow the patients across administrative boundaries.
4. Additional consultant posts were created. Stricter control of consultant contracts was proposed.
5. GP practice budgets, later termed fund-holding practices, were introduced. GPs were able to use their fund to buy care from NHS providers or private practices on a cost-effective basis.
6. Management bodies were reformed by reducing regional, district and FPC size and by putting executive and non-executive directors on the authorities. An NHS management executive was set up.
7. Better audit arrangements were instituted. Medical (peer review) audit was made compulsory throughout the NHS; and the Audit Commission was asked to audit the financial accounts of the health authorities including the Family Health Service Authority and the NHS bodies.

Like the White Paper, the legislation sought to create an internal or quasi-market in health care by effecting a separation of the purchaser and provider functions. On the purchasing side would be the district health authorities and those GPs, initially with more than 11 000 patients, who had chosen to hold their own practice budgets, as well as private patients and their insurers. On the supply side, services would be available from a variety of providers: hospitals which remained directly managed by district health authorities (by 1994 a small minority), hospitals and community units which had opted of health authority control and become self-governing NHS trusts, private and voluntary suppliers. The link between purchasers and providers operates by means of contracts or service agreements which set out prices, treatment levels and quality standards. By means of such contracts, purchasers are able to hold providers accountable for their performance.

The aims of all these changes were the stimulation of increased efficiency in the production of services through the creation of a competitive market in the NHS in which the successful providers would expand and flourish, the boundaries between the public and private sectors of health care would blur and the health authorities would be free to measure and plan for the needs of their resident populations unhampered by the domination of self-interested providers.[11]

But these aims, and methods by which a more competitive, efficient and responsive health service might be achieved, by no means commanded universal support. The publication of *Working for Patients* generated a storm of criticism from a wide variety of sources which persisted during the period when the bill was before Parliament. Given their past history of unwillingness to accept reform, it is not surprising that organisations representing the medical profession were in the vanguard of opposition. The BMA mounted a significant and costly campaign but a wide variety of other interests became enjoined with the government in 'a battle of propaganda and counter-propaganda that was remarkable for its scale and cost, for the furious intensity and acrimony of its conduct and for the levels of personal vilification to which it sometimes descended'.[11]

In essence, opposition to the government's proposals was two-fold. On the one hand it questioned the feasibility of specific proposals contained in the White Paper and the parliamentary bill. On the other, it challenged the legitimacy of introducing market principles into the health care sector and stood firm against what it saw as creeping privatisation. Common to both was 'a deep-seated fear about the long-term impact of the internal market'.[13]

Despite, or perhaps because of, the opposition mounted against its proposals, the government maintained its strong commitment to reform and adhered to a strict timetable for the introduction of change. This represented a high risk strategy for the government.

Electorally the NHS tended to be a vote winner for the Labour party. More voters, when questioned, affirmed their faith in the Labour party to maintain the principles on which it had been founded and to fund the service adequately. The introduction of more explicit market principles into the British health care system thus represented a considerable electoral risk for the Conservatives. The political consideration of a general election to be held at the latest in 1992 created the need to show success in health care reforms before that time. There was thus a heavy pressure on ministers to activate and implement the reforms speedily. When the general election did occur the Conservatives, under the new leadership of John Major, secured a fourth consecutive term in government. That outcome ensured the continuance of the NHS reforms—though Labour too had begun increasingly to use the language of the market in the early 1990s—and some further developments. These have included the standard-setting of the Patient's Charter, the re-designation of the regional health authorities as regional offices of the NHS Management Executive and the introduction of league tables for hospitals.

Each of the changes that has been introduced since the 1991 reforms highlights the nature of the health care market that has been created. In essence, it is a planned market in which the buying and selling of services operates within a carefully controlled framework of management and regulation. As such, it is in considerable contrast to the vision of the market expressed in *Working for Patients*. That document was 'the ambitious product of a political environment that preferred private to public domains, markets to bureaucracies, competition to patronage and individual choice to social equality'.[11] The language of ministerial and departmental written papers, immediately after the White Paper was published, was one of the flavour of the free market. But 'in the propaganda battle for the hearts and minds of the people'[11] this gave way to a softening of the language. Market changes were replaced by notions of better service and were expressed in more user-friendly terms. Thus 'buyers' became purchasers; 'sellers', providers; 'contracts', service agreements. 'GP budgets' became GP funds and those to whom they applied, fund-holders. 'Self-governing hospitals' became NHS hospital trusts: with an emphasis on the NHS, because the Labour party insisted on talking loudly about 'opting out of the NHS'. But, in addition, new terms were devised to describe new elements in the reform process which were never envisaged either by think-tanks or government. These were 'block contracts', an anti-market phrase by definition, and 'steady state' which really meant no change. Such changes in language designed to stem the tide of contemporary criticism, however, have themselves led to some of the major problems seen in 1994. The terminology may have altered; what, then, of the reality as the health service went to market?

Implementation

> Introducing market-like mechanisms into a planned system of health care was never going to be easy.
>
> *Wendy Ranade*[3]

Running in parallel to the national level of policy change by legislation, local plans designed to prepare for change began to develop selectively among district health authorities, hospital units and GPs. At times, such local discussion simply added to the chorus of protest. But, in addition, it also began to highlight issues of practical concern. These included the inadequacy of existing information systems, the shortness of time for the implementation of the reforms and the government's unwillingness to countenance the testing of its reforms by pilot projects. The advocacy of demonstration projects was not just a delaying tactic from a naturally suspicious and antagonistic medical profession. Throughout their training would-be practitioners are taught to be suspicious of new treatments or techniques and to assist in experimentation and clinical trial before change is accepted. In the mammoth task, as the BMA perceived it, of changing the NHS, experimentation and pilot had a sound professional rationale. In addition, it was a perspective on change which gained the support of Alain Enthoven, the American health economist, whose views on the purchaser/provider split had exercised such an impact on the nature of the government's reforms.

The government, however, proceeded without such demonstration projects and with a minimum of consultation. By mid-May 1989 Mr Clarke, whilst still denying the need for 'formalised academic monitoring or evaluation', was telling the House of Commons Social Services Select Committee that the whole reforms were experimental in nature and that lessons would be learnt and necessary changes made. The Department of Health's chief medical officer described the consultation period as 'tight'; and most opposition voices, whether political or academic, complained that the government was forcing through changes without trials and in the teeth of objection.

This especially angered the medical profession. 'What do you call a man who doesn't take medical advice?' the BMA asked rhetorically in one of its campaign posters. The answer, revealed in the photograph, was, of course, Kenneth Clarke, the Secretary of State for Health in Mrs Thatcher's government. At local level, medical opposition often crystallised around the issue of hospitals considering trust status. Consultant-led opposition seemed to indicate the growing divide 'between the sceptical and even hostile views of the doctors and the activities of many managers in preparing their applications for trust status'.[11]

Against strongly felt medical opposition, the support for the reforms both among local NHS managers and the National Association of Health Authorities (the managers' representative body) was crucial to the implementation process. Surveys carried out for the Monitoring Managed Competition research project showed a high level of support for the NHS and Community Care Act among district general managers. Though they had considerable ambivalence about the introduction of market principles into the NHS and concern at the speed with which the reforms were to be implemented, an overwhelming majority believed that the changes would make the NHS more businesslike, which was 'a good thing'. Equally, they overwhelmingly supported the separation of the purchaser and provider functions.[14] In spite of that support, however, there was a general recognition among both district and unit managers of the scale of the task and the volume of work to be undertaken in creating the conditions for the operation of an internal market. The simulation of such an internal market, code-named rubber windmill, in which 40 participants played out a variety of key professional roles in the contracting process also highlighted the difficulties and obstacles to be surmounted. In general, these included a climate of professional and public hostility, inadequate management skills for new tasks such as contracting, and insufficient or inaccurate information from the Department of Health, the NHS Management Executive and the regional health authorities. At the same time, existing services had to be maintained and, in many authorities, other major new developments were in progress.[11] All the more so is it appropriate to describe the implementation of the reform programme as 'a monumental achievement . . . effecting changes in structures, attitudes and working practices that might have hitherto been unimaginable within any time-span, least of all two years'.[11]

The speed with which the elements of the internal market have developed is one indication of the success of the government's high risk political strategy as well as of management support. In November 1989 when the NHS and Community Care Bill was published, 79 hospitals and units were actively preparing their trust applications. 57 (accounting for 12% of beds in the NHS) were successful and constituted the first wave of trusts announced just before Christmas 1990. By April 1994 there were almost 500 trusts in operation providing nearly 95% of all hospital and community health services. There has correspondingly been a dramatic decline in the number of directly managed units. What was involved in terms of operational planning is described in a study of the Bristol and Weston Health authority which was in the first wave of applications for trust status.[15]

Fund-holding general practice constitutes a second dimension of the implementation of the internal market. Initially, to qualify for consideration the patient list size had to exceed 11 000. It has subsequently been reduced first to 9000 and to 7000 from April 1993. In the first year of operation 306 practices became budget holders and, although considerable regional variations remain, 25% of the population of England were in fund-holding practices by 1993/94. Glennerster's research indicates the diversity of factors that have led GPs to become budget-holders, distinguishing between those which influenced the initial wave from those given by successive cohorts. One common motivation, however, was to be able to improve the quality of service available to their patients. 'One doctor said that rather than being a "vigorous advocate" on behalf of some of his patients, he would rather be a "purchasing advocate" for all his patients'.[16] In addition to the 'muscle' it gave them to shake up what they considered unhelpful parts of the hospital service, they also welcomed the opportunity for budgetary freedom and using savings on their budget for their practices. *En passant*, it is interesting that Mrs Thatcher required considerable persuasion by her advisers to allow this element of fund-holding to go forward. The possibility of providing more on-site services was also very attractive to the fund-holders in Glennerster's study.

All of this, however, has raised the spectre of a two-tier service with the patients of fund-holders being better served than those of non-fund-holders. But for others, the introduction of fund-holding represents the cutting edge of the reforms, not least in the challenge it presents to the traditional power centres of the NHS.

Contracting has featured in studies of the implementation of trust hospitals and fund-holding general practice. Glennerster's research indicates that local providers did not take GP contracts seriously until the practices in his sample used the threat of exit—the withdrawal of their custom—from a district health authority laboratory service which was widely considered to be unsatisfactory.[16] At a more general level, there has occurred a progressive move away from the block contract, that characterised the first year of operation, towards a more sophisticated variety of alternative contract types. But if purchasing or commissioning is to be a central stimulus to the development of the internal market in the future, a wide variety of issues, ranging from quality considerations to effective and efficient information delivery, remain to be adequately addressed.

Evaluation

It remains to be seen whether the new system will yield net benefit to the users it is designed to serve.   *Julian Le Grand and Will Bartlett*[2]

There are considerable difficulties in the way of producing an effective balance sheet of the NHS reforms. No independent, non-governmental system was established to monitor or evaluate the changes. Alongside the introduction of the internal market other changes have taken place (such as the new contract for GPs and the targets in *The Health of the Nation* and the *Patient's Charter*) which make the evaluation of the reforms *per se* more difficult. Furthermore, in the period immediately preceding the 1992 general election significant levels of additional funding were provided for the NHS. If there are recorded improvements in service provision and delivery, how far can they be attributed to extra resources rather than the introduction of planned competition?

The research which has so far been published relates to the period immediately following the introduction of the reforms. Researchers have been careful to underline the particular circumstances of the pioneers. Thus Le Grand's research indicates that hospitals applying for trust status were a largely self-selected group 'which had lower than average unit costs especially in the non-clinical departments' and which were then subject to further scrutiny and selection by the Department of Health. In consequence, he suggests that any suggestion of improved performance by trust hospitals should be treated cautiously 'as these are likely to have been those hospitals which were already performing better than the others under the old system'.[17]

The evaluation of fund-holding general practitioners suggests a more positive outcome. 'Fund-holding is probably one of the few parts of the reforms that is having the competitive efficiency effects on the hospital system that the reformers had hoped for'.[16] But since only a minority of the population are in fund-holding practices, the same and subsequent research has called into question the equity of outcomes.[18]

Neither are the criteria against which to judge the reforms unproblematic. Many of the studies so far published have used criteria such as efficiency, quality, responsiveness, choice and equity. The study by Robinson and Le Grand provides a comprehensive introduction to this type of evaluation.[19] But evaluative studies need also to address the experience of those working in the NHS and using it as patients; and to reflect the different meanings which they may give to the apparently objective criteria listed above.

Conclusion: Three Tensions

Our conclusion aims to outline three tensions which are either the result of the reforms or a reflection of pre-existing conditions in the NHS which have been made more explicit by the introduction of planned competition.

First of these is the issue of determining priorities.

Beveridge's confident belief that once the backlog of health demand had been met, the NHS would settle into a 'steady state' was invalidated almost from the start. Increasing numbers of older people, new developments in surgery and care techniques as well as rising expectations have all subsequently contributed to the situation in the NHS where demand has always exceeded the supply of available resources. In that context waiting lists have acted as an important rationing device. Clinical decisions about who to treat, by what means and over what time also constitute an important form of priority-setting.

In the post-reform NHS the district health authorities have major new responsibilities for assessing the health care needs of their population and commissioning an appropriate mix of services. But these functions continue to be carried out in the context of fixed budget constraints. Because there will always be a shortfall between matching the total needs of a population and resources 'a series of choices has to be made about which services are commissioned, in what quantities and for whom'.[20]

The issue of determining priorities, an old problem in the NHS, has been made more explicit by the reforms. Who should be involved in making such choices on behalf of population? What techniques should be employed in needs assessment? On what criteria are decisions about priorities based?

The second issue in our discussion concerns the tension between market freedom and government regulation.

We mentioned earlier how the explicit market tendencies of *Working for Patients* became transformed into the practice of managed competition. As a consequence, 'the internal market has attracted criticism from the anti-market lobby and the free marketeers in almost equal measure. There are those who see too much market and those who object that it is not market enough'.[21]

Much recent criticism has come from the latter group and has centred on the issue of regulation in all three aspects of the internal market: trust hospitals, fund-holding GPs and contracts. In each case, it has been suggested, there has been an increase in regulatory surveillance: a 'snowstorm of paper directing . . . what to do and how to do it'.[22] The reasons for such central control are not hard to find. There is the high political price of failure as well as the continuing ministerial accountability to Parliament. But 'the more administrative rules are used as proxies for market incentives, the more the control system that is the antithesis of the market is strengthened'.[21]

The chairman of the NHS Trust Federation recently suggested two strategies designed to achieve 'the chance of cost-containment through competition'. His first suggestion was for a more effective purchasing system, perhaps by open tendering for clinical services. The second concerned a changing management structure, perhaps based on the relationship between the Housing Corporation and individual housing associations, which 'will sharpen provider accountability and free us from bureaucratic, input-orientated central management'.[23] Increasing purchaser freedom and the development of more sophisticated contracts are central to the government's own strategy in attempting to take forward its changes. But how far will they resolve the tension between free market and government regulation as the internal market moves towards maturity?

Our final area of discussion concerns the tension between medical professionals, managers and consumers.

The over-bureaucratisation of the reforms, symbolised by the growth in the number of NHS managers since the reforms, has frequently been commented upon. Most recently the chairman of the BMA has suggested that the principal beneficiaries of the changes have been BMW salesmen selling or leasing high performance cars to NHS managers. The antipathy referred to earlier between consultants and managers in hospitals applying for trust status was potentially reinforced in the 1990 act by the introduction of medical audit. Despite the emphasis on medical ownership, managers were given the power to initiate the audit and some oversight of the process. As such it is easy to see how it could be perceived by the medical profession as a means of providing managerial information about 'the effectiveness and efficiency of medical care' and as 'a tool for increasing the accountability of doctors'.[24]

Important as those relationships are, it was central to the government's intention in producing *Working for Patients* that 'all the proposals ... put the needs of patients first'.[12] What, then, of patient power and consumer choice in the reformed NHS? It is difficult to avoid the conclusion that the reforms embody a limited vision of both consumers and choice.

In practice 'with the exception of an explicit promise to make it easier for patients to change GP lists, the basis of the government's argument appeared to be the neo-classical economic notion that, with the mixed market's presumed increase in operating efficiency, more services would be available to enable patients to be treated more rapidly'.[25] Nor are patients in any way able to influence the choice of services they receive. In the internal market, services are purchased on their behalf by third parties such as district health authorities or by fund-holding GPs. While ministers and officials continue to talk about extending purchaser freedom what they do not seem to have in mind is any significant extension of patient involvement in the process. To so extend consumer choice would require an end to the disparity of available information between patient and professional and may well carry implications for the GP's present role as gatekeeper to secondary care.

At a more general level, the absence of the consumer voice in the post-reform structure of the NHS was widely commented upon. If the wishes of local people were to be taken more seriously into account, critics suggested, it might have been expected that the proposals would have contained an extended role for community health councils or district health authorities.[26] In the event neither occurred. Issues of democratic accountability in the interests of working for patients, however, continue to be advocated at the level both of locality and national policy-making.[3]

If the health care system can more effectively work for patients by greater involvement in purchasing decisions and by structures of democratic representativeness, a third view suggests that consumer choice is only possible in a fully fledged competitive market. In such an environment 'consumer choice would be based, not on government promise, but on that personal power to inflict economic pain on unsatisfactory producers which consumer payment alone can bring'.[27] Yet, 'the greatest irony is that the vast majority of people are paying in taxes the full cost of the services they receive'.[27] Since they have already surrendered their potential buying power to the government via taxation they have also surrendered their ability and freedom to choose.

Those examples, indicating the different ways of working for patients, illustrate how decisions about health care continue to be value-laden and to be inescapably set within an ideological and political context. In that and many other respects the post-1991 NHS has remarkable similarities to what preceded it. But it also suggests that 'the 1991 reforms look like the beginning, not the end of a process of change'.[16]

References

1. Thatcher, M. (1989). Foreword. *Working for Patients*, HMSO, London.
2. Le Grand, J. and Bartlett, W. (eds) (1993). *Quasi-Markets and Social Policy*, Macmillan, Basingstoke.
3. Ranade, W. (1994). *A Future for the NHS?*, Longman, London.
4. Moore, J. Secretary of State for Health (October 1987). Conservative Party Conference, London.
5. Green, D.G. (1988). *Everyone a Private Patient*, IEA, London.
6. Pirie, M. and Butler, E. (1987). *Health Management Unit*, Adam Smith Institute, London.
7. Goldsmith, M. and Pirie, M. (1988). *Managing Better Health*, Adam Smith Institute, London.
8. Goldsmith, M. and Willets, D. (1988). *Managed Health Care: A New System for a Better Health Service*, Centre for Policy Studies, London.
9. Willets, D. and Goldsmith, M. (1988). *A Mixed Economy for Health Care: More Spending. Same Taxes*, Centre for Policy Studies, London.
10. Enthoven, A.C. (1985). *Reflections on the Management of the National Health Service*, Nuffield Provinical Hospitals Trust, London.
11. Butler, J. (1992). *Patients, Policies and Politics*, Open University Press, Buckingham.
12. *Working for Patients*. (1989). CM555, HMSO, London.
13. Butler, J. (1993). A case study in the National Health Service: working for patients. In, *Markets and Managers*, ed. by P. Taylor-Gooby and R. Lawson, Open University Press, Buckingham.
14. Appleby, J. *et al.* (1994). Monitoring managed competition. In, *Evaluating the NHS Reforms*, ed. by R. Robinson and J. Le Grand, King's Fund Institute, London.
15. Bartlett, W. and Harrison, L. (1993). Quasi-markets and the National Health Service reforms. In, *Quasi-Markets and Social Policy*, ed. by J. Le Grand and W. Bartlett, Macmillan, Basingstoke.
16. Glennerster, H. *et al.* (1994). GP fundholding: wild card or winning hand? In, *Evaluating the NHS Reforms*, ed. by R. Robinson and J. Le Grand, King's Fund Institute, London.
17. Bartlett, W. and Le Grand, J. (1994). The performance of Trusts. In, *Evaluating the NHS Reforms*, ed. by R. Robinson and J. Le Grand, King's Fund Institute, London.
18. *Fund-holding and Access to Hospital Care*. (1994). Association of Community Health Councils, London.
19. Robinson, R. and Le Grand, J. (1994). *Evaluating the NHS Reforms*, King's Fund Institute, London.
20. Robinson, R. (1993). Purchasing, priorities and rationing. In, *Health Care UK 1992/3*, ed. by A. Harrison, King's Fund Institute, London.
21. Hughes, D. (1993). Health policy: letting the market work? In, *Social Policy Review 5*, ed. by R. Page and J. Baldock, Social Policy Association, Canterbury.
22. Butler, E. (1994). A market future for NHS purchasing and supply. In, *Unhealthy Competition*, ed. by E. Butler, Adam Smith Institute, London.
23. McNichol, M. (1994). Innovation and entrepreneurship in NHS services. In,

Unhealthy Competition, ed. by E. Butler, Adam Smith Institute, London.

24. Kerrison, S., Packwood, T. and Buxton, M. (1994). Monitoring medical audit. In, *Evaluating the NHS Reforms*, ed. by R. Robinson and J. Le Grand, King's Fund Institute, London.

25. Saltman, R.B. and Von Otter, C. (1992). *Planned Markets and Public Competition*, Open University Press, Buckingham.

26. Neuberger, J. (1990). A consumer's view. In, *The NHS Reforms: Whatever Happened to Consumer Choice?*, ed. by D.G. Green, IEA, London.

27. Green, D.G. (1990). A missed opportunity. In, *The NHS Reforms: Whatever Happened to Consumer Choice?*, ed. by D.G. Green, IEA, London.

Chapter 5

From Evolution to Revolution: Restructuring the New Zealand Health System

Toni Ashton

Department of Community Health, School of Medicine, University of Auckland, New Zealand

Introduction

On budget night, 30 July 1991, the New Zealand government announced a radical restructuring of all publicly funded health services.[1] These reforms, which were implemented on 1 July 1993, have been highly contentious. Supporters consider that the changes will make services more transparent, improve efficiency, reduce waiting lists and increase consumer choice.[1] Opponents argue that the system is costly and as yet uncertain and unproven.[2] They emphasise the need for co-operation within the health sector rather than competition, and for evolutionary change rather than revolution. While business people are generally in favour of the changes many health professionals remain strongly opposed to them. A survey of nurses, for example, reported that 82% of respondents were generally opposed to the reforms.[3]

This chapter discusses some issues underlying the reforms and some implications of the changes from an economic perspective. The chapter begins with a review of the background to and reasons for the changes. The main features of the proposals are then described. This is followed by a discussion of the theoretical and ideological issues underlying the reforms. Finally, some of the issues raised by the changes themselves are discussed.

Reforming Health Care: The Philosophy and Practice of International Health Reform.
Edited by D. Seedhouse. © 1995 John Wiley & Sons Ltd.

The Reasons for Change

The government's share of total health expenditure has been steadily declining in recent years. Nevertheless, in 1993 public funds still accounted for just over 75% of total health expenditure.[4] The government also provides most hospital services in New Zealand although the majority of primary health services are privately owned.

In the years immediately prior to the reforms, the New Zealand health system had already undergone a period of considerable change. Between 1983 and 1989, 14 area health boards were established, the role of these boards being to provide hospital services, public health services, and some community services for the people of their region from a population-based global budget. In 1988, a rather cumbersome triumvirate system of hospital management by doctor, nurse and administrator was replaced by general management. In 1989, a set of national health goals and targets was developed to establish spending priorities and the boards were required to draw up strategic and business plans for all of their services.[5] Accountability of the boards was established through a contract with the Minister of Health based on these plans.

As a result of these changes, the area health boards began to operate in a more business-like fashion and there appeared to be some evidence of productivity improvements.[6] But waiting lists and waiting times remained unacceptably long.[1] Budget constraints were often manifested in ageing equipment and poor maintenance. Moreover, productivity gains were not universal and some area health boards were getting into debt. It was also argued that, because area health boards owned their own facilities, there was no incentive for them to contract with more cost-effective providers if they existed.[1]

Another problem arose from the fact that most primary care was funded separately by the central government on a fee-for-service basis. This meant that, unlike area health board budgets, public funding for primary care was open-ended. Patient user charges already applied to general practice services and pharmaceuticals. Nevertheless, the government was concerned that primary care expenditure was increasing steadily and could not be controlled directly.[1] The separate funding for primary and secondary care also meant that patient care was poorly integrated and some cost-shifting occurred.

In 1986, the funding of primary care services was reviewed and recommendations made.[7] However no action was taken. Then in 1988, a task force reported on hospital and related services but again no changes were made.[8] Finally, in February 1991 soon after a change of government, a third task force was appointed to review the whole spectrum of publicly funded health services. The recommendations of this group were not published separately but instead were used as the basis for that part of the government's annual budget of 31 July 1991 which became known as 'The Green and White Paper'.[1] The two colours of the cover indicated a desire for the document to be regarded in part as a discussion (green) paper and in part as a policy (white) paper. In fact, it very soon became apparent that the paper was more white than green, there being little or no room for any discussion or submissions from interested parties prior to the introduction of legislation to implement the reforms.[9]

The Main Features of the Reforms

The central feature of the restructuring was the splitting of the purchaser and provider roles previously carried out by the area health boards. The 14 boards were replaced by four regional health authorities (RHAs) whose role is to assess the health service requirements of their populations and to purchase services as necessary from the most cost-effective providers. The RHAs are responsible for purchasing primary health care (which was previously centrally funded) as well as secondary, tertiary and community services. A committee, known as the National Advisory Committee on Core Health and Disability Support Services (NACCHDS), was charged with the task of defining explicitly those services that RHAs are obliged to offer to the people of their regions. A separate national authority, the Public Health Commission, was established to plan and purchase public health services for the total population.

The hospital and community services previously owned by the 14 area health boards were reorganised into 23 Crown Health Enterprises (CHEs). They act as independent businesses with appointed boards of directors, and are required to pay both taxes and dividends to the government. Links between the RHAs and providers are established through legally-binding contracts. The basic premise is that, by simulating some of the features of a competitive market, both purchasers and providers will face incentives which encourage greater efficiency in service provision.

In the 1991 Green and White Paper it was proposed that, once RHAs were fully established, people would be given the opportunity to take their share of government funding to a non-government alternative purchaser (a health care plan), the amount of their entitlement reflecting their level of risk. Thus the intention was to introduce competition not only amongst providers but also at the purchasing level. While this proposal has been shelved for the time being, the legislation covering the reforms does make provision for alternative purchasing agents, subject to government recognition.[9]

Theoretical and Ideological Underpinnings

During the second half of the 1980s, the dominant school of economic thought in New Zealand, as elsewhere, fell into the general category of monetarism. Interestingly, unlike most other countries, in New Zealand these policies of macro-economic restraint and micro-economic restructuring were first introduced by a Labour government although the National (conservative) government elected in 1991 continued in much the same vein. Policies included balanced government budgets, a stripping back and restructuring of the Welfare State (including increased user charges for education and health), and the corporatisation and privatisation of many government enterprises.

The ideology underpinning these policies includes a general belief in the superiority of markets over governments, of competition over co-operation, and of self-reliance over community responsibility. The abandonment of any commitment to an egalitarian society by the New Zealand government has been discussed by Boston and Dalziel[10] who note that:

> . . . important values such as human dignity, distributive justice, and social cohesion, have been given second place to the pursuit of efficiency, self-reliance, a fiscal balance, and a more limited state.

The introduction of more business-like arrangements and greater competition into the health services is in accord with these economic and social trends.

The relevance of the competitive market model to health services has been the subject of a long-standing debate amongst economists. Proponents of the market view hold that health services are no different from other services in terms of the expected responses to market mechanisms.[11,12] Therefore, strengthening market mechanisms should improve the efficiency of health services and so achieve greater value for money. Those of the opposing view, articulated in the New Zealand context by the Wellington Health Action Committee,[2] consider that market theory has limited application to health services. Reasons for this include the difficulty of measuring the output of health services; problems of asymmetry of information between patients and health professionals, and hence the need for health professionals to make decisions on behalf of patients; and the judgement that everyone should have access to health services regardless of their ability to pay.

As well as the prevailing market liberal school of economic thought, the health reforms reflect a number of more specific influences. The splitting of purchaser and provider follows the broad recommendations made in the 1988 Taskforce on Hospitals and Related Services[8] which had been chaired by Alan Gibbs, a businessman who was a close friend of the Minister of Finance. A second report prepared in 1990 for the Business Round Table—a right-wing think-tank comprising the chief executives of large industrial companies—was also influential. In this report, P. Danzon, a visiting professor from the US, outlined a path for the corporatisation and eventual privatisation of both the delivery and funding of health services in New Zealand.[11] The corporatisation of health service provision in July 1993 closely parallels the first step of the three-step process proposed by Danzon. Some commentators have argued that, in spite of government assurances to the contrary, the direction of health policy is now clearly heading along the path towards full privatisation of provision and funding.[2]

The reforms also follow the general direction of the National Health Service (NHS) in the UK. But the New Zealand reforms are far more radical in a number of ways, especially in terms of the autonomy of all hospitals, the integration of funding for primary and secondary services, and the potential to introduce competing purchasers. These features more closely reflect the Dekker proposals for the reform of health services in The Netherlands. In that country however, the reform process, which commenced in 1989, is progressing only slowly and is not expected to be completed until 1995 or later.

Some Implications of the Reforms

The one point upon which there appears to be general agreement is that the new system will cost a lot more to administer. Fourteen area health boards have been replaced by four RHAs and 23 CHEs, each of which has its own management structure and board of directors. Large investments are required in information technology and specialised expertise to design, negotiate, monitor and enforce the contracts. The crucial question is whether the potential efficiency gains will outweigh these additional costs. The expectation of policy makers was clearly that significant net savings could be achieved. In spite of deficiencies in the supporting data, the Gibbs and Danzon reports both argued that 'huge gains . . . are possible in the hospital sector'[8] and 'large potential gains are beyond doubt'.[11] This belief was reiterated repeatedly during the reform process. For example, Peter Troughton, a businessman appointed to oversee the corporatisation of public hospitals, predicted efficiency gains of up to 30%, while the Minister of Health, Bill Birch, said that he expected the new service to generate between NZ$270 million and $540 million* to purchase new and extra services.[13]

The key to potential efficiency gains lies in the contracting process. In theory, competitive bidding for contracts should ensure that RHAs purchase services from the most cost-effective providers, while providers have an incentive to produce at least cost so as to secure contracts and maximise their financial returns. But there are a number of reasons why, in practice, the process may produce less efficient outcomes than expected.

The incentive for providers to produce efficiently depends in part upon the degree of competition that providers face. In New Zealand the small size and wide dispersity of the population means that there is only one provider of health services in many localities. Even in urban areas, economies of scale and the need for specialist expertise discourage the existence of more than one provider of some services. Thus RHAs have little choice but to contract with incumbent providers, at least in the short term. This absence of competitive pressure as an incentive for efficiency may be offset by the fact that the CHEs will be monitored by a central government agency and provided with feedback about how their performance compares with other CHEs. The open publication of these performance indicators would provide a more powerful incentive towards efficiency but this option has been rejected by the government in the interests of commercial sensitivity.

To encourage cost-minimisation and to secure a return on public assets, the original draft legislation required CHEs to be 'as profitable and efficient as comparable businesses that are not owned by the Crown'.[14] The wording of this clause was subsequently changed following widespread objections in public submissions on the legislation. CHEs are now required to provide services 'while operating as a successful and efficient business'.[9] However, while the letter of the law was altered, the spirit remains much the same.

The requirement for CHEs to be successful financially raises important

---

* NZ$1.00 = 41p sterling, or US$0.64 (January 1995)

questions about the underlying ethics of health service providers and about the compatibility of financial targets with social objectives. As well as the requirement to be successful and efficient, the legislation also requires each CHE to 'exhibit a sense of social responsibility by having regard to the interests of the community in which it operates'.[9] There are many instances where these two objectives could conflict. CHEs could, for example, increase their surpluses by selecting those patients who are likely to cost least, or by admitting private paying patients ahead of publicly funded (i.e. non-paying) patients. The inevitable result of this would be that access to services is restricted for those in greatest need.

Although competition is likely to be limited, the reforms do open up opportunities for private providers, some of whom were previously denied access to public funds, to bid for contracts. However many private organisations which have the potential to compete with CHEs (especially for elective surgical procedures) are non-profit organisations which pay neither dividends nor taxes. This puts CHEs at a competitive disadvantage. Public hospitals are further disadvantaged by the fact that their clientele have, historically at least, generally been sicker and poorer (and hence more costly) than the clientele of private hospitals, few of which cater for serious complications or major trauma. Furthermore, in order to ensure the provision of less-profitable services, the Minister may require a CHE to provide a service for 'a reasonable price . . . but any dispute as to such a price shall not entitle the enterprise to withhold those services'.[9] This not only disadvantages CHEs but also compromises their profitability.

In the first six months of operation, the CHEs recorded combined operating losses of almost NZ$100 million.[15] Moreover it was announced that profits were not expected for another three years. Accumulated debt almost doubled from $700 million taken over from the area health boards to $1.26 billion. The government argued that these losses could not be attributed to the new system. Rather the new system revealed for the first time just how much it was actually costing to supply health services:

> One of the major benefits of the restructuring to date has been the improvement in the information available to make more accurate assessment of revenue needs for Crown Health Enterprises.[6]

In response to this apparent need for additional funding, the government announced a $405 million injection of funds into the health sector over a three-year period. While efficiency gains were still expected to permeate through the system over time, it was obvious that the level of savings originally predicted was unlikely to be achieved. The expected level of efficiency gains was therefore scaled down significantly to 5%.[13]

In purchasing services, a central problem that RHAs face is that they have less information than providers about the services. In particular, they have less information about the production process and cost structures. This problem is in part offset by the fact that the RHAs, being the dominant purchaser in their regions, enjoy considerable bargaining power. Nevertheless, RHAs may find it difficult to evaluate prices, especially where there are few providers and no obvious pricing yardsticks. Even where there are many providers, costs vary significantly due to factors such as (dis)economies of scale, costs of provision in urban and rural areas, availability of voluntary labour for some private providers, and so on. In this environment, RHAs are likely to find it difficult to determine whether price differences are due to internal efficiencies, or real differences in cost structures. Information about production processes such as mix of the workforce and technological inputs is zealously guarded by providers on the grounds of commercial sensitivity.

An associated problem is the difficulty of measuring quality of service. The specification of indicators of quality that are both meaningful and measurable has proved elusive for many services and little work is being undertaken on the impact of services on health outcomes. Because of the imbalance of information between RHAs and providers about production processes, RHAs may be tempted to define quality requirements—to the extent that they can be specified—according to existing production methods. But this discourages innovation and may constrain potential efficiency gains. A study in the US found that, contrary to expectations, competitive bidding for services led to a lack of innovation because contracts were won by those providers who could meet certain quality standards set by the purchaser.[17]

A feature of the new system that appears to be inconsistent with the market liberal view which underlies the reforms is the central prescription of a set of core health services which must be purchased by the RHAs. Justification given for this explicit definition of core services was 'to protect the level of health services and hold RHAs . . . accountable', and to 'get better value for scarce resources and seek to limit the growth of medical expenditure'.[1] However the intention is for RHAs to be customer-driven and to purchase those services which best meet the needs and preferences of the people of their region. The central prescription of core services limits the ability of RHAs to adjust their purchasing patterns in response to consumer needs. This suggests that, contrary to the rhetoric used to support the reforms, an efficient allocation of resources is not expected to be achieved automatically through the strengthening of market forces, even if competing purchasers are introduced.

The attempt to define core health services raises a host of other economic, ethical and political questions which are outside the scope of this paper. At a more practical level, the attempt is meeting some major technical barriers, not the least of which is the dearth of information about the quantity, quality, use and cost of existing services. Initially, the committee concentrated on doing a stock-take of existing services and identifying broad service priority areas.[18,19] In the first year, RHAs were given a directive simply to roll-over the range and volume of existing services and try to smooth out differences in access to these services as indicated by national utilisation rates.[20] Unfortunately the use of regional comparisons to establish some sort of ideal utilisation rate only tells us what is: it says nothing about what ought to be, either in terms of economic efficiency or social preferences. While the approach to be taken by the core committee has not been stated explicitly as it has in The Netherlands and Oregon, the committee was appointed 'to represent the views of the community to the Government'. This seems to imply that some kind of community perspective is intended, as it was (in different forms) in the above two projects.

The requirement to roll-over existing services was removed in the 1994/95 RHA policy guidelines so that RHAs now have greater freedom to adjust their purchasing policy, subject to national standards and service priorities.[21] However it remains unclear just where the boundaries of responsibility and decision-making lie between the core services committee, representing the views of the community nationwide, and the RHAs, representing the populations of their regions.

One argument that has been advanced in favour of the purchaser/provider split is that the contracting process should improve the accountability of providers by making explicit the quantity and quality of services supplied. Interestingly, under the previous system accountability was stronger amongst area health boards which were both purchasers and providers (but which had contracts with the Minister of Health) than it was amongst primary health care providers where the purchasing and providing roles were split. In fact, somewhat contradictorily, the lack of accountability of primary care providers was itself advanced as one of the major reasons for reform! Clearly it is not the split itself which secures accountability but the nature of the contracts, and whether these contracts can be monitored and enforced satisfactorily and at reasonable cost. Enforcement through the legal system is likely to be costly. It is also likely to be inappropriate in cases where courts lack the commercial and medical expertise required to review decisions.[22]

Questions are also being raised about the accountability of the RHAs to taxpayers. Each RHA will be required to '. . . on a regular basis consult in regard to its intentions relating to the purchase of services'.[9] However the nature of the consultation process has not been specified. Moreover, neither RHA board meetings nor contracts between RHAs and providers are open for public scrutiny. Thus it is not clear as yet just how accountability will be achieved.

Conclusion

The New Zealand health reforms represent a departure from the egalitarian philosophy that has traditionally underpinned health service provision in this country. The reforms are based upon an ideological commitment to competitive markets rather than upon any clear empirical evidence that the changes will achieve greater value for money, thereby improving the health status of New Zealanders. The process of translating the theory into practice has proved costly, difficult and controversial and many details have yet to be decided. The morale of many in the health sector has been undermined by the uncertainty created by the changes. Moreover, the public health service in New Zealand was once based upon a wide measure of co-operation and many are now critical of its replacement by competition.[2]

If nothing else, the reforms have generated widespread debate and raised important questions about priorities in health services. They have also encouraged providers to examine their methods of provision, to consider how and where efficiencies might be achieved, and to set up appropriate information systems. Whether any efficiency gains will be sufficient to outweigh the additional costs of the new system remains to be seen.

References

1. Upton, S. (1991). *Your Health and the Public Health*, A Statement of Government Health Policy by the Minister of Health, Wellington.
2. Wellington Health Action Committee (1992). *Health Reforms: a Second Opinion*. A Comprehensive Critique by Leading Health Commentators, Wellington.
3. Wills, D.J. (1991). A survey of nurses' views on the latest health service 'reforms', *New Zealand Nursing Forum* 19(4), 6–7.
4. Muthumala, D. and McKendry, C. (1994). *Health Expenditure Trends in New Zealand: Update to 1993*, Department of Health, Wellington.
5. Clarke, H. (1989). *A New Relationship: Introducing the New Interface Between the Government and the Public Health Sector*, Report by the Labour Minister of Health.
6. The Treasury (1990). *Performance of the Health System*, unpublished internal report, Wellington.
7. Report of the Health Benefits Review (1986). *Choices for Health Care*, Wellington.
8. Report of the Hospital and Related Services Taskforce (1988). *Unshackling the Hospitals*, Wellington.
9. *Health and Disability Services Act* (1993).
10. Boston, J. and Dalziel, P. (1992). *The Decent Society?* Oxford University Press, Oxford.
11. Danzon, P. and CS First Boston NZ Limited (1990). *Options for Health Care in New Zealand*, Report for the New Zealand Business Round Table.
12. Logan, J., Green, D.G. and Woodfield, A. (1989). *Healthy Competitions*, Centre for Independent Studies Policy Monograph 14. Australia.
13. A $405m tourniquet won't stop the bleeding. *New Zealand Herald* (1994). 5 March, p. 8.
14. *Health and Disability Services Bill* (1992).
15. Health entities slump deeper into the red. *New Zealand Herald* (1994). 18 March, p. 5.
16. East, P. Minister of Crown Health Enterprises, (1994) *Additional Funding will assure future of nation's public health enterprises*. Media Statement, March 2nd.
17. Schlesinger, M., Dorwart, R. and Pulice, R. (1986). Competitive bidding and states' purchase of services, *Journal of Policy Analysis and Management* 5(20), 245–263.
18. National Advisory Committee on Core Health and Disability Support Services (1992). *Core Health and Disability Support Services for 1993/94*. First Report to Minister of Health, Wellington, New Zealand.
19. National Advisory Committee on Core Health and Disability Support Services (1993). *Core Services for 1994/95* Second Report to Minister of Health, Wellington, New Zealand.
20. Upton, S. (1992). *Policy Guidelines to Regional Health Authorities*, Statement by the Minister of Health.
21. Shipley, J. (1994). *1994/95 Policy Guidelines to Regional Health Authorities*, Statement by the Minister of Health.
22. Chen, M. (1993). Judicial Review under the Health and Disability Services Act 1993, *Public Sector* 16(4), 220–223.

Chapter 6

Choosing Core Health Services in The Netherlands

Henk A.M.J. ten Have

Department of Ethics, Philosophy and History of Medicine, Catholic University of Nijmegen, The Netherlands

Introduction

The current debate on health care resource allocation in The Netherlands is being conducted in a social context in which two values—solidarity and equity—are generally accepted as fundamental.[1-4] Since World War II the guiding principles of all Dutch governments, conservative or progressive, have been 'equality of access to health care' and 'solidarity in sharing the financial burden proportionate to income'. These principles are reflected in the health care system. Access to health care is not limited, either by geography or financial considerations. Since The Netherlands is a small country, there is no problem of distance. Physicians and hospitals are distributed fairly evenly throughout the country. Practically no one is without health care insurance; two-thirds of the population (below a specific income level) are covered by mandatory national health care insurance, while the others are privately insured. For those insured through the state (not including the privately insured) the burdens of paying for health care are distributed evenly (since the premiums are proportional to income).

Towards the end of the 1970s an increasing tension was felt between the values of equity and solidarity. The foundational nature of these values was not questioned but the ensuing political debate concentrated upon their implication and range. Over the last 25 years, the relative investment of the national product in health care has risen markedly from approximately 4% to 9%. Per capita health care expenditure has shown an average annual growth of 0.6% since 1980 (if the price-level of 1980 is taken as the standard).[5] Such increases have occurred in spite of cost-contraining measures (such as the introduction of

Reforming Health Care: The Philosophy and Practice of International Health Reform.
Edited by D. Seedhouse. © 1995 John Wiley & Sons Ltd.

budgeting systems in hospitals and the reduction of specialists' salaries) applied to various points of the health care system.

Searching for Fundamentals

In The Netherlands the main issue has not been the question of how to distribute scarce resources, but how to find a (new) balance between individual interests and the general welfare.[6] Although there is a stronger tendency now to focus on financial aspects, it is important to realise that the problem of resource allocation is usually discussed within a broader framework than the economic one, since proper deliberation must also involve inquiry into the political and philosophical foundations of the Welfare State.

For three reasons, developing a more fundamental approach became politically relevant, especially for government, political parties and health care advisory bodies, in the 1980s and 1990s.

1. A Welfare State which emphasises equal access and solidarity has its price. The population's willingness to support the collective financing of health care services is lessening, but compensating for increasing costs requires higher taxes and premiums. Roughly 36% of each individual's personal income goes into taxes and premiums for social security and health care. If continued, this policy will further erode general willingness to apply the principle of solidarity—already under pressure through increased emphasis on individual responsibility in health care—to the financing of health care.
2. The government has introduced a series of proposals to reorganise the health care system to introduce a system of basic health insurance for all, thereby changing the differentiated system of compulsory and voluntary insurances. Although the desirability of national health insurance is not really disputed, there is political controversy over the type and number of services to be funded in an elementary insurance system, for it is obvious that the new basic package will not cover all presently insured services. The controversy essentially concerns the inadequacy of the principle of equal access in times of scarcity, since the principle provides little or no guidance on which rationing policies should be applied.
3. Changes in the pattern of demand and supply in health care also necessitate the reconsideration of health care policy. The population is ageing: the proportion of those over 65 will increase by 20%, that over 80 by a third by the year 2005.[8] As a result, there will be an increasing disease load and more chronic and degenerative disorders. Demand for health care facilities (and particularly for chronic care facilities) is bound to increase. At the same time, scientific and technological change in medicine will continue to attract public attention, and fund the demand and expectation for new diagnostic and treatment interventions.

Three options are available to reduce pressure on the health care system: (1)

allocate more money for health care; (2) become more efficient; (3) make explicit choices about care.

The first option has been ruled out by government. Higher taxation or insurance rates are politically unrealistic and other social goals such as education and a good environment also compete for collective resources. Therefore, according to the Cabinet, the volume of care in 1990–4 may increase by a maximum of 1% per year.

The second option, to increase efficiency, has received much attention over the past decade. It was not considered ethical to make choices in health care and deny some patients care so long as money was being wasted by inefficient care. Many projects have started to deliver care efficiently, and to make use of diagnostic tests and treatment schedules; and much more yet can be done to reduce wastage of resources. However, it is estimated that even maximum efficiency will not lead to more than 15% reduction of the costs of important health care services.[9] That implies that increasing efficiency can delay the need to make choices but it cannot prevent the necessity for choice in the longer run. Therefore, the third option—making choices in health care—is the most realistic one. But then the question is: how should such choices be made?

Basic Health Care Needs and the Concept of Health

In August 1990 the State Secretary for Welfare, Health and Cultural Affairs installed a Committee for Choices in Health Care. Its task was to develop strategies for making choices between existing and new possibilities in health care, particularly with regard to the package of necessary services to be included in the new mandatory insurance system. Three main questions appeared on the Committee's agenda: (1) why make choices? (2) between what do we have to choose? (3) how should we make choices? The Committee was also explicitly invited to initiate and stimulate a public discussion (as in Oregon, for example), about the relative necessity of services available in the current health care system.

The Committee published its report in November 1991. It strongly argued that choices in health care are unavoidable and desirable. Even if more resources were to be available for health care, explicit choices would still be necessary. Most important, the Committee proposed a set of guidelines for making fair choices.

The starting-point for the Committee's argument is the proposition that everyone who needs health care must be able to obtain it. However, equal access to health care should not be determined by demands but needs. In order to have a just distribution of services, it is not important that all services are equally accessible, what is crucial is what services are accessible. Not every health care service is equally relevant for maintaining or restoring health. Thus it is important to identify 'basic care', 'essential services' or 'core health services' focused on basic health care needs in contradistinction to individual preferences, demands or wants. 'Relevant needs' should be distinguished from all the things we can come to demand or want. In his theory of health care needs, Daniels argues that needs are distinct in relation to their object, namely health.[10] The concept of health is therefore the most appropriate standard for characterising health care needs, since it is argued that health enables persons to maintain a normal range of opportunities to realise their life plans in a given society. Since it and not health care services as such are 'basic' or 'essential', the Committee prefers the expression 'necessary' because it implies a relationship between the particular kind of care or service with a particular goal ('necessary for what?').

Strategies for Making Choices

The Committee defines health in general terms as the ability to function normally. However, 'normal function' can be approached from three different perspectives:

1. *The individual approach.* Here, health is related to autonomy and self-determination. It is the 'balance between what a person wants and what a person can achieve'.[11] Defined as such, health can vary according to individual preferences. But in this case no distinction is possible between basic needs and preferences; what is a basic need for one will not be for another. This approach therefore is not helpful in determining on a societal level what the 'necessary care' is that should be accessible to all. Even if through a democratic decision-making process (such as in Oregon) the largest common denominator or the smallest common multiplier of individual demands could be determined, we would lack criteria to identify necessary care.[11]
2. *The medical professional approach.* Typically the medical profession defines health as 'the absence of disease'. This approach is defended by Daniels. He interprets health as 'normal species-typical function', disease is defined as 'deviation from the natural functional organisation of a typical member of a species',[12] and the basic functions of the human species are survival and reproduction. Health care is most necessary where it prevents or removes dangers to life and enhances normal biological function. On this approach, 'necessary care' may be distinguished according to the severity of illness and this was proposed as a criterion by a Norwegian committee in 1987.[13] Nevertheless, this approach has a tendency to neglect the psychosocial functioning of individuals. It is also questionable whether normal species-typical functioning can be defined regardless of the social circumstances.
3. *The community-oriented approach.* In this approach, preferred by the Committee, health is regarded as the ability of every member of society to participate in social life. Health care is necessary 'when it enables an individual to share, maintain and if possible to improve his/her life together with other members of the community'.[14] 'Crucial' care is what the community thinks is necessary from the point of view of the patient. This approach is not utilitarian because what is considered to be in the interests of the community is dependent on its social values and norms. Every community exists by presupposing a normative, deontological framework defining the

meaning of its interests. In Dutch society at least three normative presuppositions define the communal perspective: (1) the fundamental equality of persons (established in the Constitution); (2) the fundamental need for protection of human life (endorsed in international conventions); and (3) the principle of solidarity (expressed in the organisation and structure of social systems, particularly the health care system).

Within this normative framework the Committee has distinguished three categories of necessary care: (1) facilities which guarantee care for those members of society who cannot care for themselves (e.g. nursing home care, psychogeriatric care for the mentally handicapped); (2) facilities aimed at maintaining or restoring the ability to participate in social activities when such ability is acutely endangered (e.g. emergency medical care, care for premature babies, prevention of infectious diseases, centres for acute psychiatric patients); (3) care depending on the extent and seriousness of the disease. From a community-oriented perspective, the first category is more important than the second or the third, and the second more important than the third.

Follow-up

The proposals of the Committee are intended to start a broad public debate on health care services. The Ministry of Health has allocated a substantial budget (several million guilders) to increase the number of participants in this discussion. Indeed, especially among organisations of women, patients, handicapped and elderly, many initiatives and activities have been started. However, the political debate so far has been disappointing. The Cabinet response (in June 1992) focused primarily on promoting appropriate care, giving a major role to health care professionals in defining standards of care and treatment protocols.[15] It seems therefore that in the political arena explicit choices in health care are not yet made, notwithstanding the intentions that led to setting up the Committee. This is an unfortunate situation since the medical profession has been given the task to decide how to cope with scarce resources, but the most the profession can do is ameliorate the consequences, it cannot really solve the problems. Without explicit decision-making at the macro level the basic principle of solidarity will further erode. Solidarity implies that the autonomous individual learns to recognise that his own interests are best served by promoting the common good. Introducing a uniform package of core health services, without making distinctions between 'needs' provided for by the state, and 'wants' provided for by people themselves, and without clarifying criteria to make such distinctions through broad communal debates, is a recipe for losing control over increasing health care costs.

What is needed is a policy which guarantees equal access to services which provide for communally agreed necessary care as well as special protection of vulnerable groups within the community in order to maintain equality of result and opportunity. The Committee report provides a strategy for linking the idea of a basic package of health care with the concept of necessary care available to all. Now, or in the near future, health care politicians must take up the challenge.[16]

References

1. Boot, J.M. (1990). Health policy in The Netherlands. *BioLaw* **2**(35), 1619–1622.
2. Have, H.A.M.J. ten and Keasberry, H.J. (1992). Equity and solidarity: The context of health care in The Netherlands. *Journal of Medicine and Philosophy* **17**, 463–477.
3. Verkerk, M. (1990). Solidarity and health policy. *BioLaw* **2**(35), 1631–1636.
4. Wachter, M.A.M. de (1988). Ethics and health policy in The Netherlands. In, *Health Care Systems*, ed. by H.M. Sass and R.U. Massey, Kluwer, Dordrecht, pp. 97–116.
5. Government Committee on Choices in Health Care (1992). *Choices in Health Care*, Zoetermeer, p. 41.
6. Have, H.A.M.J. ten (1988). Ethics and economics in health care: a medical philosopher's view. In, *Medical Ethics and Economics in Health Care*, ed. by G. Mooney and A. McGuire, Oxford University Press, Oxford, pp. 23–39.
7. Have, H.A.M.J. ten (1990). Health and responsibility as policy tools. *BioLaw* **2**(35), 1623–1630.
8. Government Committee on Choices in Health Care (1992). *Choices in Health Care*, Zoetermeer, p. 35.
9. Van de Ven, W.P.M.M. *et al.* (1988). Doelmatigheid in de gezondheidszorg: een miljardenkwestie. *Nederlands Tijdschrift voor Geneeskunde* **132**, 1623.
10. Daniels, N. (1985). *Just Health Care*, Cambridge University Press, Cambridge (Mass).
11. Government Committee on Choices in Health Care (1992). *Choices in Health Care*, Zoetermeer, p. 51.
12. Daniels, N. (1985). *Just Health Care*, Cambridge University Press, Cambridge (Mass), p. 28.
13. Royal Norwegian Ministry of Health and Social Affairs (1990). *Health Plan 2000*, Oslo.
14. Government Committee on Choices in Health Care (1992). *Choices in Health Care*, Zoetermeer, p. 54.
15. Tweede Kamer der Staten-Generaal (1992). 22393, nr 20, *Modernisering zorgesector Weloverwogen verder*, Sdu Uitgeverij, Den Haag.
16. The Committee's report is available from: Ministry of Welfare, Health and Cultural Affairs, P O Box 5406, 2280 HK Rijswijk, The Netherlands.

Chapter 7

Reforming Health Care in South Africa

Michael A. Simpson

Department of Psychiatry, Medical University of Southern Africa, and Institute for Mental Health Policy Development, Pretoria, South Africa

Apartheid and Health

Health care policy making is *never* apolitical, and the extent to which state funds can be diverted to the care and feeding of ideological fantasies should not be underestimated. Before it is possible to understand any potential health policy developments in South Africa one must comprehend the extent to which a profoundly sick society was carefully, almost obsessively, created there. South Africa is not a normal society within which the usual pathologies occur. Apartheid and health were[1] 'incompatible and mutually exclusive' and apartheid was such a massive programme of social engineering that much pathology in this nation continues to be the direct or indirect result of government policy.

South African apartheid is an archetypal illustration of the impact of politics on health care and development. The South African government, especially since 1945, pursued policies to monopolise power and redistribute wealth to its Afrikaner Nationalist supporters (i.e. to a minority of the white minority). The most charitable interpretation of the facts is that successive members of that government and its bureaucracies designed and administered policies with reckless disregard for the health and lives of the great majority of the population, and in irresponsible ignorance of the likely (often inevitable) consequences of their actions. The more radical interpretation, again entirely consistent with the facts, is that much of the misery was a desired or at least an acceptable, expected, and planned result of sophisticated and cynical policies. Whatever the truth, accountability by public officials for their actions and decisions (let alone the results of these actions and decisions) was a tradition wholly foreign to the South African regime.

Since the new health policies currently being devised for the newly democratic

---

Reforming Health Care: The Philosophy and Practice of International Health Reform.
Edited by D. Seedhouse. © 1995 John Wiley & Sons Ltd.

South Africa are in good part reactions to the iniquities and inequities of past policies, they are best understood in relation to what has gone before.

A Word of Caution

One must be very cautious about accepting the figures quoted by the apologists for apartheid (a group which includes much of the South African medical establishment). Politicians have interfered with the accuracy of health statistics. For example, after 1976, various artificially and politically defined areas were called 'homelands' and given artificial independence, and various sham states were declared to exist. These areas were then ignored in official statistics about the extent of disease in South Africa. And since they generally showed especially high incidences of major illness, the South African health statistics appeared to improve, at a stroke; and the new, manipulated figures, were often quoted as evidence for the health benefits of the apartheid system. For example, by excluding the Transkei, where 6% of the population suffered from tuberculosis (TB), the incidence of TB in 'South Africa' dropped instantly, even though all these tubercular patients were still living there.

While official statistics were often highly inaccurate, the necessary steps were not taken to improve them, for to do so would suggest a worse health status than was politically convenient. A survey in KwaZulu,[2] found that 8 in 1000 people had TB, when official notification data claimed only 1.8 per 1000. Furthermore, it is a fact that 15–30 000 children in South Africa die of starvation or malnutrition-related illnesses each year, but accurate official figures were not kept.

The uncritical use of racial descriptors in South African medical literature has been criticised.[3] However, it remains important to use them to describe the effects of a health system that was based on such a classification in order to retain the ability to recognise such effects and to work for the reduction of discrimination. In recent years departments of the old regime stopped gathering and issuing statistics on a racial basis on the composition of staff: not as a step towards non-racialism, but to obscure the immensely high proportion of white and male staff they maintained. A study of the reliability of mortality data in Johannesburg[4] found substantial under-reporting of deaths in official statistics, especially among the aged and infants. Taking this into account would have raised the infant mortality rate from 14.1 to 19.1 per 1000 live births.

Early Historical Distortion of Health and Health Care

Until early modern times the Boers placed great stock in folk remedies, such as goat dung for measles, and wolf dung for sore throat. When the four colonies joined as provinces in the Union of South Africa in 1910, the new constitution made no mention of health care except to give responsibility for administration of hospitals to the provinces. Only in 1919, after the great influenza epidemic, did the Public Health Act create a Ministry of Public Health.[5]

In 1928, the Loram Commission was set up to look into the training needs of African doctors, and rejected proposals for a shorter training and lower entrance qualifications for African doctors, advising full equality with the white medical profession. Appointed to 'inquire into the training of natives in medicine and public health' it commented drily that:

> It cannot be denied that at present there are hordes of natives in many centres who have little chance of medical treatment, and the untreated sick become a menace to the community. Indeed, not just a menace but a double menace to South Africa. Firstly, there is the immediate danger of the spread of infection and contagious diseases from areas where they may be said to be practically endemic. Secondly, there is the economic danger of the deterioration and eventual failure of the labour supply.

One can see the unconscious racism. Being black, the untreated did not constitute 'the community', but rather a commodity which was a potential threat to the community. The perceived problem was not that suffering and death would result, but that 'the labour supply' might fail.

It is important to recognise that, although racist distortions of health and health care and the routine abuse of human rights reached maximum efficiency under successive Nationalist regimes following 1948, their roots lay deep in white politics, in legislation begun under British rule and even earlier. The 1913 Land Act established 'reserves', where families were expected to rely on subsistence farming, to provide a source for low-paid migrant labour. The 1923 Urban Areas Act began clearing 'mixed' urban areas, creating separate 'locations' for black Africans. It restricted the number of Blacks in urban areas, requiring them to carry a 'pass', and those unable to find jobs had to leave within 14 days.

The Nationalists serially tightened legislation and ruthlessly enforced it. Africans not born in an urban area were not allowed to reside there unless they had lived there continuously for 15 years or worked for the same employer for 10 years. The maximum time allowed in an urban area to seek work was dropped from 14 days to 72 hours. Passes had to be carried at all times. The Group Areas Act of 1950 enforced the creation of separate residential areas for Coloureds and Indians, as well as Africans, and separate local government structures.

Afrikaner ideologists later justified the crimes against humanity that typified the regime on the basis of the need to withstand a 'Communist total onslaught'. Apartheid was also justified on the ground that it protected people from the effects of soulless capitalism.[6] Such earnest opposition to capital seems to have been strictly limited to capital in the hands of others: Afrikaner capital was regarded as free from all unwholesome side-effects. The Draconian 1950 Suppression of Communism Act defined as communism any doctrine or scheme which encouraged 'feelings of hostility between the European and non-European races', by which ironic definition, every South African government prior to 1994 has been communist.

The National Health Services Commission, 1942–1944

> What is wrong with our present health services? . . . Under the present system the majority of people are deprived of the advantages of modern medical services. The service rendered is determined not by the individual's susceptibility to disease, but by his ability to pay. Members of the medical profession are compelled, under the present system, to practise for gain and are said to have a vested interest in disease.

One of the great ironies of public health history is that South Africa had a splendid plan for a national health service in 1944, a plan with wide international influence at the time; but the opportunity for implementing it was squandered shortly before the introduction of apartheid. The words quoted, though they would provide an entirely accurate contemporary summation of South African health care, were used in 1942 by Dr H Gluckman, Member of Parliament, proposing a commission of inquiry which became the National Health Services Commission of that year, under his chairmanship. It reported in 1944.

With uncommon vision, it found an unacceptable incidence of disease, blamed largely on social and economic conditions.

> Vast numbers of people in this country do not earn enough to purchase the minimum of food, shelter and clothing to maintain themselves in health.

It recognised the unco-ordinated, ill-planned deficiences of existing services and proposed a system to provide good quality 'free' health care to all. Despite wide acclaim and government adoption, the main recommendations were never implemented. The United Party government under Smuts essentially ignored it; subsequent Nationalist governments were busy designing and establishing apartheid, so non-discriminatory health care was never seriously considered.

The Gluckman Commission correctly identified the 'almost monotonous repetition of divided and incoordinated control in every branch of the health services in South Africa', a situation arising from careless inattention by government, but which later became required and imposed by governmental policy. At that time, nationwide, there was one hospital bed for every 304 Whites, yet only one for every 1198 Blacks. In Cape Town, there was one doctor for every 308 white people; in Zululand one for every 22 000; and in Northern Transvaal, one for every 30 000. Eighty two per cent of specialists were concentrated in the four major cities.

The Commission recognised that merely providing more 'doctoring' would not really improve public health without great improvements in nutrition, housing and health education. It proposed a National Health Service in which 'all personal services should be made available to all, and shall be a national instead of an individual responsibility', and provided free of direct charge, funded by a National Health Tax, based on the principle 'from each according to his means, to each according to his need'.

The state would take over all hospitals from the provinces which would supply environmental health services including sanitation and clean water. The system would be based on Community Health Centres, one for each 10 000–

30 000 people, staffed by a multi-disciplinary team, including health visitors to link the centres to the community. Private practice would be phased out. Many more health workers of different categories would be trained. The 1942–44 Commission advised equal opportunity in the NHS, 'and equal pay for men and women performing work of the same nature'.

Most notably, it said 'we wish to state emphatically that we are opposed to any selection which discriminates between one race and another'.

Six months later, the government accepted the recommendations with two reservations: control of curative medical services should remain with the provinces, and the system would be introduced 'in a series of measures, not in a single step'. This effectively prevented proper planning and co-ordination of curative care and enabled that government and its successors to fail to introduce any of the other recommendations.

The Medical Association of South Africa (consistently a powerful and highly conservative lobby over the years) strongly opposed much of the Report, especially the concept of state-employed doctors and the idea of free medical care to all: it demanded a means test, insisting that care for the poor should remain a charity and not a right.

Dr Gluckman was made Minister of Health in 1945, and until his removal in 1948 when the Nationalist government accelerated the building of apartheid, he had seen to the construction of some 40 health centres. An Institute of Family and Community Medicine opened in Durban in 1949, but as there was no consistent or sufficient funding, integration or administrative support, the centres could not function, and the National Health Service was aborted. Over the next 20 years the original health centres were closed or transferred to ordinary clinic functions.

Apartheid and the Promotion of the 'Illfare' State

From 1948, the efforts of the Nationalist governments to secure white Afrikaner hegemony, regardless of the impact on the health of the nation, took precedence. Only after the 1976–77 township revolts did the government consider slight changes in health care, as a potentially safe area within which to provide a simulation of reform. Following the 1977 Health Act and later pronouncements, increased emphasis was placed on 'preventive health', and even on community health centres (in fact a parody of the Gluckman system); changes that were more apparent in propaganda announcements than in real practice. And this in the following context: by 1970, in de Beer's summary, Whites, only 17% of the population, earned 72% of the income. Africans, 70% of the population, earned only 19% of the income. Between 1960 and 1970 the gross difference between white and African wages had increased by 76%. The division of land (13% to the 'Bantu', 87% to Whites) was described by Prime Minister Vorster as 'decreed by history'.

Job reservation policies restricted entry by Blacks into all jobs with good pay; no effective black trade union activity was allowed. Black workers, previously largely confined to 'locations' (where a pool of workers were 'located' when not required) were moved to 'townships', deliberately far from white suburbs and from their jobs. This required long and expensive commuting (many black workers paying 10–20% of their wages for such transport), but such dormitory areas were more easily policed and controlled. Others were pressed towards artificial 'homelands' in distant rural areas.

In 1968, the state decided to stop building houses in the urban townships, which were administered by undemocratic Bantu Affairs Administration Boards, and dominantly financed by profits on the sale of alcoholic liquor controlled by the Boards (in some cases this was as much as 80% of the budget). Thus, any improvement in 'health amenities' such as clean water and electricity, depended on increasing rent (the Boards owned the houses) and increasing liquor sales: hardly a structure destined to improve health. As late as the 1980s, the government instructed Boards to cut back on black housing. Rural poverty was an inevitable and irresistible force driving rural inhabitants to the cities, so there was an inexorable increase in 'illegal' city dwellers, who increasingly had to live in shacks lacking all proper amenities.

Government propaganda proclaimed rising wages of black workers; while ignoring rising unemployment (often over 20% in a nation with no significant welfare provision), and ignoring the rising cost of living. De Beer,[2] for instance, cites a survey showing that the average real income of people in Soweto fell by an average of 18.5% between 1978 and 1980, while rents increased by over 100% and electricity rates soared by 400% between May and October 1980 alone. It was estimated that half of Soweto households lived below the absolute poverty line: although Soweto residents were better placed for access to jobs than most township dwellers.

De Beer[2] has summarised the extent of health hazards at work, and the comprehensive neglect of industrial health hazards by government and industry. Some European companies, unwilling to meet European safety standards, moved to South Africa, where the regulations were more limited, the authorities more understanding, and workers more hampered by state policy in their attempts to protect themselves.

Inequality in the Provision of Health Services, and the Costs of Apartheid

There has been a poor collection and late reporting of health information; but available data has consistently shown gross racial discrepancies. The 1991 population was 37.7 million growing at an average of 2.5% per annum; 75% were Blacks, 13% Whites, 9% 'Coloureds', and 3% Indian).[7] Data for 1985, published in 1992,[8] showed the infant mortality rate in Blacks (probably underestimated, as registration of births and deaths has not been compulsory for Africans) was 73 per 1000 live births for males, and 68 for females; while in Whites it was 11 for males, and 7 for females. The 1989 maternal mortality rate was 8 per 100 000 for Whites, and more than 58 per 100 000 for Blacks.

Adult mortality rates (estimated as the chance of a 15 year-old dying before reaching the age of 60) were 42.8% for black males, and 29.4% for black females; 21.87% for white males, and 11.5% for white females. Life expectancy at birth was 55 for black males and 61 for black females, 68 and 76 for white males and females, respectively. Being born black was the single greatest risk factor for almost all varieties of health hazard (except for the diseases of affluence, access to which was strictly limited).

Infant mortality rates per 1000 population in 1990, according to Slabber,[9] were 9 for Whites, 12 for 'Asians', 35 for 'Coloureds', and 52 for Blacks. Of notified cases of TB (by no means all cases, and certainly underestimating black cases), the incidence per 100 000 was 17 for Whites, 61 for Asians, 608 for 'Coloureds', and 213 for Blacks.

According to van Rensburg and Fourie,[10] per capita expenditure on health in 1987 was: R591.11 for Whites, R356.24 for Asians, R340.16 for Coloureds, R137.84 for Blacks within the statistically truncated South Africa (RSA), and R54.74 for Blacks in the 'homelands'. At current exchange rates, that last figure would be less than £10 sterling per annum. All health-relevant figures show the same consistent discriminations. For hospital beds, the ratio was 1:61 Whites, 1:505 Indians, 1:346 Coloureds, 1:337 Blacks (RSA), and 1:417 Blacks in the homelands. As regards practising doctors, the ratios ranged from 1:282 Whites, 1:661 Indians, 1:10 284 Coloureds, 1:53 543 Blacks (RSA), and an unreliable 1:8333 for homeland Blacks is quoted. The distribution of dentists ranges from 5:10 000 for Whites, through 1.3:10 000 for Indians, 0.25:10 000 for Coloureds, to 0.005:10 000 Blacks. About 90% of all dentists are white.

It has not been uncommon to find hospital bed occupancy rates of 150% or higher. I have known wards with an average of three patients per nominal bed: one in the bed (more, in the case of children), one lying on the floor under the bed or in the corridor, and one waiting on the grass outside for a death or discharge to allow access to space inside. Zwarenstein and Price[11] found overall bed ratios of 150 Whites per bed: 130 in urban areas, 260 for rural Whites. While the overall ratio for non-Whites was 260 per bed, this varied from 150 in urban areas, to 300 in 'homeland' areas, and 460 in other rural areas.[7]

Costs

The costs of apartheid itself, the expense of maintaining manifold non-productive bureaucracies, multiplication of facilities, etc., have never been adequately calculated. In 1989, it was estimated that in one of the smaller provinces, R37 million a year was wasted maintaining apartheid in the teaching hospitals alone. In the 1980s, a decade after state promises to 'rationalise' the public service, South Africa contained 11 presidents, prime ministers or chief ministers; five ministers of national security, 14 ministers of finance, 11 ministers of the interior, and, at its peak, 18 ministers of health. Above these overt structures, there was also a secretive State Security Council, not answerable to 'democratic' structures, and with nine area command structures, 60 regional or sub-structures, 448 local or mini-structures, each with sub-committees.

Old Wine in New Bottles: Strategies for Avoiding Change

Typical of misleading propaganda seeking to disguise the realities of the persistent failure to provide properly for the needs of the majority, was a report issued by the South African government for overseas use which said:

> The Bantu, generally speaking, are not yet what is termed a developed people . . . Persuading the Bantu peoples of South Africa to accept modern medicine has been a big task, involving a painstaking campaign ... It has not merely been a question of bringing the medicine, the vaccines or the mobile units to the Bantu people, or indeed, bringing the Bantu peoples to the doctors, the nurses and the hospitals. The real struggle has been against ignorance, superstition, mistrust, fear and witch-doctors. Gradually, however, the Bantu is being weaned away from the centuries-old superstitions and belief in witch-doctors, and the future is hopeful.[12]

A recurrent ploy has been the highly publicised announcement of new health plans or policies, without any significant consequent change in actual practices, nor any improvement in results. In 1977 a new Health Act was proclaimed, followed by supposed implementation details in a Health Services Facilities Plan, both of which were ambiguous documents. In line with more sophisticated propaganda skills, they dripped with the terms currently in vogue internationally: fashionably praising community health, preventive medicine, decentralisation, community participation, attention to the needs of the poor, health promotion and 'the elimination of the causes of ill-health', and deprecating high-technology and hospital-based care. They even proposed a network of community health centres. Gluckman reborn!

But there was no substantial or significant change in actual health systems, practices or budgets. Few health centres were built; it was cheaper and less troublesome to re-name some existing or ordinary clinics and give the impression of compliance. Spending on preventive health care soared from 2% of the health budget to some 3%. No effective central health authority was created. Instead, a progressive splintering of authority, control, and planning capacity was assiduously pursued. Two new advisory bodies: a Health Policy Council and a Health Matters Advisory Committee, were created. Neither ever distinguished itself by the quality or independence of its advice; both were perpetually dominated by government appointees and appointees of government appointees; resolutely undemocratic, opaque, isolated from relevant communities, and without demonstrable beneficial impact on health.

The health plan increased the endemic lack of co-ordination of health care. It ensured that the foundations of health, such as water, food, sanitation, and housing, remained the responsibility of multiple departments, agencies and sectors. Basic level health care, it airily stated 'will be provided by voluntary health organisations' which were to 'play an active supplementary role in the rendering of health services'.

Yet such organisations received no particular encouragement or assistance to embark on such roles, not even effective tax breaks for donors. Community participation, as de Beer[2] wryly points out, seemed largely to mean that unfavoured communities would have to look after themselves when and where the state avoided its responsibilities.

In the late 1970s, the state realised the attractions of encouraging the private sector to take over as much health care as possible, recognising that this would reduce potential claims on the state. In the 1980s, a wave of Thatcherism overran government health planners: privatisation became *de rigueur*,[13–16] fervently promoted by a few, accomplished surf-riders on the waves of social trends—advice peddlers unblemished by any actual experience of the process they were selling.

As the 1978 *Guide to the Health Act* commented:

> It is not the aim or objective of the legislation to diminish private practice in any manner. On the contrary, the more people placed in the position to afford the services of private practitioners, the less will be the burden on the state.

Care was taken to ensure that community health centres should not compete with private practitioners. There was concerted effort by the government to deflect its responsibilities for provision of health care back onto the individual, and to use extra 'perks' to encourage key personnel who might resist privatisation to modify their resistance.

The private hospital sector[17] is substantial: 48.9% of all hospitals, with 29% of all beds. Apart from charity, welfare, and industrial hospitals; a national TB charity, SANTA, has 22 hospitals. An unusual and controversial phenomenon is the 'contractor hospital': privately owned facilities, run for profit, but which have contracted with the state (usually on a fixed fee per patient per day basis) to provide care for some types of patient, notably long-term psychiatric and TB patients. There are 23 such hospitals, dominated by the Lifecare corporation (formerly known as the Smith-Mitchell group).

Further Planned Damage to Health Care

Beyond 1992, health services were further damaged by thoughtless government budget cuts and a programme of indiscriminately offering early retirement to public service staff, causing 'unplanned, undirected and unselective cuts in health care'.[18] Grossly clumsy labour relations typified the regime's health administration.[19] In 1993, the Public Service Labour Relations Act, forced through Parliament against fierce opposition, removed the right to normal professional bargaining on wages and working conditions.[19,20] In 1992, a prolonged strike by NEHAWU, a dominant hospital workers' union, which appeared to be deliberately provoked and extended by intransigent bureaucrats, caused further suffering.

Fresh harm to the system was inflicted by the government's decision to allow 'limited' private practice (of 20% of the working week) in academic centres; failing to provide an acceptable salary package,[21] and ignoring the dangers of this move, which has damaged patient care and teaching. Irresponsibly failing to evaluate the effects of the diktat, or to modify it in the light of its obvious faults, was grossly neglectful. Having tried by this means to buy the support of senior academics, the Ministry then discovered that it had to extend the same privilege to all doctors in the public employ, and to nurses, physiotherapists, and others.

Scientific Chauvinism

During the years of increasing isolation and unacknowledged shame about apartheid, it was especially unfortunate that the world's first heart transplant happened to occur in South Africa, as it fostered publicity-seeking high-technology chauvinism that distorted perceptions and realities within health care. The *South African Medical Journal*, for example, has shown obsessive concern about the need for provision of heart transplantation, one of the least relevant issues in terms of national needs, devoting more editorial space in recent years to that topic than to any other single treatment modality.[22-26]

Odell and Brink[24] typify the triumphal and bellicose scientism that still vigorously defends the monumental irrelevancy of the first Groote Schuur heart transplant:

> It demonstrated to the surprised world our expertise in medicine. The flag of that first transplant was waved vigorously in the faces of our critics as an example of the excellent standard of medical care practised in South Africa.

The degree of misunderstanding required to see the luxury transplants as representing a standard of national medical excellence, when thousands of children were dying from lack of access to simple oral rehydration is awe-inspiring.

Similarly, a major professor of surgery made the extraordinarily revealing comment that medical schools faced a dilemma in the choice between:

> on the one hand unswerving dedication to the pursuit of excellence, and on the other the obligation to the needs of our society as a whole.[27]

He seemed genuinely unaware that this need be no dilemma, and that medicine that is not devoted to its obligation to the needs of its society as a whole is never ever excellent. His implied definition of excellence as exclusively constituted by the medicine practised by glittering super-specialist transplant surgeons in very expensive hospitals with extremely expensive equipment is typical of attitudes that endanger public health. One can be more unswervingly devoted to the pursuit of excellence in rural primary care than in transplanting baboon livers.[16] True excellence lies in doing whatever needs to be done, as well as it can possibly be done, and wherever it needs to be done.

Constraints on Health Policy Planning in South Africa

In South Africa we do not have adequate dynamic data on the distribution of health personnel and the factors influencing such dispersal,[28] nor do we have adequate morbidity and mortality data.[8,29-31] There is inadequate information on health resource allocation and use;[11] and on the causes of sickness and death.[31] Such data as is published is usually long out of date.

Basic information systems are non-existent or incompetent: none of the state health services, to date, has been able to provide data on the costs of procedures and services; hardly any usable data are accessible from the private sector. The national Director-General of Health has been unable to provide data on health expenditure of the 'homelands', even though such expenditure came from the central government budget. Hospital superintendents and health administrators, national and provincial, are rarely adequately trained or skilled, and often recruited from those who had failed to succeed in any other area of health care provision. Rehabilitation services, convalescent facilities, day hospitals, and similar basic components of health care are almost non-existent in large areas of the nation, and poorly developed in even the most privileged areas. Endemic political and criminal violence places a continuing load on health care facilities. With responsibility for many services which in other countries would be provided by the state, hived off to non-governmental organisations (NGOs) and community organisations, the degree of fragmentation is increased.

There is rapid population growth, at a rate of almost 3% per annum, and a doubling of the population is projected for the next 25–30 years. Improvement of health care will be limited unless the economy can recover from its present state of stagnation. A complete change of administrative culture is needed. There has never been competent planning, control of activities or budgets, skilled management, or democratic consultation of health workers, let alone patients.

The Process and Nature of Change

In the run-up to the first democratic elections in 1994, in which all parties were for the first time able to compete and were asked to declare their policies, there seemed very little at issue—at least as regards rhetoric and vocabulary—between the various major political parties and interest groups, on their declared health policies. In the prolonged process of the 'negotiated revolution' that led to political transition, the politicians too often and for too long avoided detailed discussion of the details of *how* such ideals would be achieved, for fear of encountering a jarring lack of unanimity.

In South Africa, despite the first world glitter of the facilities for the privileged minority (now defined financially rather than racially, but with very similar effect), the people's health can still be substantially improved by spending *outside* the traditional health budget. Experience in Britain and other countries showed that by far the greatest drop in infant mortality rates—in death rates from rheumatic fever, tuberculosis, and other scourges—occurred in the century before the availability of chemotherapy, and from improvements which resulted from spending on housing, santitation, water supplies, education, and employment. The deliberate underdevelopment and the carefully planned damage of the apartheid era left much of the South African population still living in conditions that would make those of the poorest areas of Dickensian London seem privileged. This unfortunate situation does, however, mean that one can anticipate a similarly significant health bonus to accrue from general national development.

The ANC National Health Plan for South Africa

The *South African Medical Journal*'s new editor welcomed the penultimate draft of the ANC National Health Plan (NHP)[32] with an extraordinarily snide comment, politically and morally naive to an astonishing degree, opining with regard to the data the plan provided about the deliberately discriminatory resource allocation and socio-economic circumstances that 'apartheid receiv(es) the obligatory tongue-lashing'.

The editorial shows, rather more clearly, the obligatory tongue-lashing meted out by supporters of the old regime to those who, much more noticeably than Dr Ncayiyana, opposed and criticised the massive damage to the health of the community inflicted by apartheid. The NHP would have to have been ethically and scientifically blind to a peculiar degree had it failed to record the major political reality shaping South African life, resources, and health care.

The Main Features of the ANC National Health Plan (NHP) 1994

The plan is committed to the review of all legislation, organisations, and institutions related to health, to ensure that their emphasis is on health and not merely on medical care; on team-work and the equal importance of all health workers, 'recognising that the most important component of the health system is the community'; on ensuring mechanisms are created to enable 'effective community participation, involvement, and control'; and on introducing management structures for efficiency and compassion, 'ensuring respect for human rights and accountability' to users. These are laudable aims, almost perfectly the opposite of those which guided the old system. The challenge will be to find effective means of achieving them in routine practice.

The NHP was drawn up with vastly more consultation than any previous South African government policy document: but, given the history of arrogant and non-consultative government, which only consulted selected members of the ruling caste who were bound to agree with any proposals, it was not difficult to exceed that dismal record. But there was, still, far less broad and democratic consultation than was needed; contributions were often unacknowledged; and the process remained far too susceptible to influence by a priviliged few in the new elite, from politically correct units with little or no experience of health care delivery or administration, and little record of close community consultation. The process has often been grossly sloppy. For instance, an essential drug list is proposed, and has supposedly been worked on for years, but not a single draft has been released for comment or discussion among interested parties. The process of further formulation of health policy needs urgently to follow its own advice and become more transparent and democratic.

This early problem points to an area of inevitable difficulty needing prompt attention. Democracy—or even the simulation of democracy—is cumbersome. As was once said of socialism, it takes up too many evenings. During this period of emergence from extreme repression and authoritarianism there has been such an intense and urgent need for consultation of so many parties on so many themes (reconstruction and development, health, education, housing, employment, justice, and a host of other urgent problem areas) that community leaders and representative groups have had difficulty in scheduling the host of meetings and invitations.

The NHP wrestles, as expected, with pragmatic goals for health. It realistically recognises that improvement in health will occur:

> mainly through the achievement of equitable social and economic development such as the level of employment, the standards of education, and the provision of housing, clean water, sanitation and electricity.

One has some doubts about the place of electricity (and, in another proposal, telephones) quite so high in the list of priorities: these facilities deliver less health dividends, are less essential to living a healthy life; and the cost of the universal provision of these amenities in very remote rural areas will divert scarce resources from more urgent needs.

Much thinking about health policy has been mesmerised, for decades, by the World Health Organisation's definition of health as 'a state of complete physical, mental and social well-being and not merely the absence of disease or infirmity': a state of bliss which most people approximate or imitate briefly, if at all, only at the height of orgasm, and thus rather difficult to achieve as the routine product of a health service.[33] The NHP says:

> Every person has the right to achieve optimal health, and it is the responsibility of the state to provide the conditions to achieve this.

Functional definitions of 'optimal' and 'conditions' are needed. An earlier draft (ANC, 1992) asserted that:

> Access to health care is a basic human right . . . This right will be incorporated in the Constitution and the Bill of Rights and will be enforced by law.

The institution of a constitutional court with the duty and authority to decide on whether such stated rights are duly provided by the health care system can be expected to lead to challenging debates.

Even the US Constitution only guarantees the freedom to *pursue* happiness, not necessarily the achievement of constant or routine happines. I believe that everyone has the right to pursue the highest level of health they personally can and choose to attain; and that it is the responsibility of the state to guarantee that the health of individuals and communities will not be impaired by the actions or inactions of others, including the state, and that access to basic health care should not be limited by poverty, or by factors related to racial, ethnic, religious, political, or gender or sexual preference issues. A right to health, such as is often described, is no more logically defensible nor practically enforceable, than a right to wisdom, or to beauty. We are differentially endowed by nature with the necessary substrate for approaching each of these desirable states: our right, surely, is that we should not, unreasonably nor with prejudice, be impeded from seeking to achieve them.

The NHP calls for a 'single comprehensive, equitable and integrated national health system (NHS)' which will 'co-ordinate all aspects of both public and private health care delivery and will be accountable to the people of South Africa through democratic structures'. Authority over, responsibility for, and control of funds will be decentralised to the lowest possible level compatible with rational planning and maintenance of quality; with administration being divided among local, district, provincial, and national authorities. This favouring of devolution of power towards local communities is understandable, but in fact it will require an even larger bureaucracy than the previous splintered system; and co-ordination, promotion of efficiency and avoidance of duplication will be difficult.

First contact with the NHS will be via clinics or health centres, and independent general practitioners. The emphasis is fiercely on the 'primary health care approach' as defined in the Declaration of Alma Ata: it states, uncompromisingly, that primary health care 'is the best possible form of health care for everyone, rich and poor alike, in any society'. It proposes to heal the former split between health and social services/welfare; and proposes 'a social security net'; but leaves the details and mechanisms vague and open to continuing discussion.

The NHP analysis of the existing situation[7] is very similar to that presented above. The NHP is committed to reduce inequalities, especially in deprived communities. Perhaps due to energetic lobbying, it emphasises the absolute needs of women and children, sometimes minimising those of men and the elderly. There is a committed emphasis on maternal and child health, and free provision of health care services in the public sector to all children under six was the first part of the NHP to be implemented after the April 1994 election. Free antenatal, delivery and postnatal care was also considered a primary step.

An intersectoral development committee is proposed, to ensure collaboration between the actions and policies of the many sectors of governmental and private activity relevant to health.

Specific health policies stated in the NHP contain a policy towards human immunodeficiency virus (HIV) and acquired immune deficiency syndrome (AIDS) that is generally unexceptional by international standards, but a considerable improvement on the disastrous neglect typical of the previous government. Amongst other responses, it provides for HIV counselling and support services at all community health centres, 'easy access to abortion should they choose it' for women infected with HIV who become pregnant; recording of the number of all HIV cases, though HIV/AIDS will not be notifiable; and no restriction on the sale or distribution of condoms (the previous government allowed extraordinary restrictions at times), and the removal of all import duties on them. Despite expert advice, the plan does not provide explicitly for the necessary palliative care for the large numbers of people who are dying and will die of AIDS: but states that 'the compassionate care of HIV infected people must be guaranteed', in the context of 'a chronic illness requiring on-going care to maintain the quality of life of those infected'.

It further declares that 'laws and regulations discriminating explicitly or implicitly (against HIV-infected people) will be reviewed and repealed' which could have an interesting impact on currently discriminatory regulations in medical insurance and other insurance company provisions, which act against people with HIV infection.

A National Commission of Health Technology (sic) is to focus on appropriate health technology, maintain a rational policy and regulate the importation of expensive technologies (viewing highly specialised technologies and equipment as national resources 'whether in the public or private sector').

After the needs of the elderly were ignored in earlier drafts, a rather feeble and vague section is now included, but it makes no definitive contribution to the great needs of this much neglected group. Only in the opening 'Executive Summary' (an odd sort of summary, as very significant items 'summarised' within it appear nowhere else in the NHP) does it state that 'free health care will be provided in the public sector for children under six, pregnant and nursing mothers, the elderly, the disabled and certain categories of the chronically ill'.

Among other revelations in this interesting summary are: the introduction of a Charter of Patients Rights (again, no general discussion of such a Charter has been mounted, and no draft has been circulated); a Commission of Inquiry to review the current crisis in medical aids/medical insurance, and 'to consider alternatives such as a national health insurance'; a Commission of Inquiry to make recommendations on conditions of service of health workers; a commitment to health personnel education being multi-disciplinary, gender sensitive, problem-oriented and community-based, with 'a number of fast-track training programmes to be introduced for unspecified 'categories of urgently needed personnel'; and an increase of user fees at public hospitals for insured patients so as to ensure full cost recovery, with the hospitals being allowed to retain a proportion of this revenue to improve the quality of their services.

The drug policy, as mentioned, is still not even half-baked, but some clear trends are visible. 'At registration, cost-effectiveness will influence . . . initial price', and 'complete registration will depend on agreement being reached on this initial price'. Generic prescribing and generic substitution, will be encouraged, as will therapeutic protocols. The total failure of those engaged on advising the ANC on drug policy to provide any drafts of the sort of protocols they envisage, the range of the proposed 'essential drug list' in the public sector, or the means by which they would seek to encourage a strong local pharmaceutical industry, has provided no confidence in their competence or efficiency.

There is a strong emphasis on health promotion. The new government's first budget ignored the proposed special tobacco tax, apparently in response to the usual vigorous lobbying by this very powerful South African industry; though new and strong warnings on cigarette packs have been proposed. Cadres of community workers are envisaged, earnestly promoting health, although little evidence has been offered that such fashionable intervention actually produces much measurable improvement in standards of health: the main benefit is likely to be simply the side-effect of job creation and the provision of local employment opportunities.

Although mental health is a declared priority, policy in this field is still vague and non-specific, and ill-developed: there are few useful details, and heavy reliance on 'fostering liaison and co-operation', and 'supporting', 'improving', and 'extending' various services. Despite the large scale of the needs of survivors of violence and civil conflict[34,35] there's merely a one-line statement favouring support and development of services for those so affected.

Provision is made for patient access to traditional healers and to promote more collaboration with allopathic/Western practitioners; encouraging the control and registration of traditional medicine by an accepted body to promote this profession and eliminate harmful practices.

Although there is a lack of sufficient detail in all areas, there is enough to promote the lively national debate that needs to be encouraged. However there is little sign of any provision for the open debates we were assured would follow. It is a welcome novelty for any party in South African politics to publish a reasonably detailed health plan at all, let alone shortly before an election. Only the formerly ruling National Party revealed an alternative policy on health prior to the first democratic elections (mainly platitudes and anodynes, and strikingly similar in broad outline to the ANC policy); none of the many other political parties who took part in the 1994 elections stated any coherent or comprehensive health policy at that time, or managed any intelligible or useful comment on health matters during the campaigns. The first draft of the Pan Africanist Congress (PAC) policy began to circulate for discussion only during and after the election, and is discussed below.

The PAC Policy

The policy is very enthusiastic, proclaiming far more areas as of high priority than are likely to be dealt with seriously. But erring in the direction of excess ambition to achieve equitable health care is a novel and welcome error by comparison with the smug complacency of the preceding decades of government.

There are detailed 'organograms' of the relationship between the many new administrative structures proposed, and attempts to allocate functions between the various parts. Several commentators have expressed concern that the structure is bureaucratically heavy, especially for a country in which the previous regime developed a system in which a peculiarly large proportion of the white population worked for state or para-statal administrations.

Ambitious targets for achieving some of the identified health care priorities are outlined; some specific, e.g. measles immunisation 'coverage to 80% by end 1995, 90% by end 1997'; some very broad, e.g. 'improve health services in rural areas'.

In April 1994, a first draft of a health policy for the PAC[36] began to circulate. Far more politically explicit, its analysis of the existing system and its weaknesses is consistent with what has been discussed above; and I will thus comment only on its more unusual features. It offers an even more detailed and thoughtful analysis of the existing problems and constraints. The basic premises of the PAC national health policy match those of the ANC plan, but are expressed, for example, as a need to 'decolonise' and to 'restructure health services to redistribute health resources to the historically dispossessed African people'.

Like the ANC, it proposes to provide a 'basic health package', without specifying, even in draft form, the likely contents of such a package. Among its short-term goals, for 'immediate provision', it proposes an 'independent national network to promote the health service, audit its performance and deal with complaints'; and in several sections refreshingly emphasises evaluation and assessment of outcomes. Surprisingly, among its long-term goals (for the next 10 years) is 'expansion of the state capability for secondary and tertiary health care including cardiovascular surgery, joint replacement and transplantation surgery', which is considerably at variance with any other published priorities.

It has a broader vision of involvement in health policy development and health promotion, including trade unions, the media, commerce and industry, and 'the sports world'. There are intriguing statements such as: 'the food, alcohol, tobacco, drug, motor and arms industry shall be in line with the best interests of the health of the nation'.

The PAC document commendably starts to suggest specific statements of patient rights and health service standards. Here, as in some other sections (such as a jarringly unco-ordinated appearance of 'hospital trusts'), one senses a clear influence of recent documents from the British health service. The attitude toward multi-national drug companies in its drug policy is surprisingly accommodating, when considered in relation to the party's otherwise radical policies.

The PAC policy effectively recognises an area insufficiently faced by the ANC plan, and wisely specifies the need for training at all levels of health services administration in health policy planning, the management of promotive health programmes, assessment of individual and community health needs, and also in communication and public relations skills. Both plans overlook the equally important need to provide information and skills training for the community and its chosen representatives, to ensure that community participation is effective rather than merely a token pretence.

Conclusion

To some readers I may seem to have been somewhat strident in this critique of the South African health care system and its recent history. Burdened with direct experience and detailed knowledge of the cruelties of the repressive era from which we are only beginning to emerge, and convinced that the mealy-mouthed re-writing of the facts of South Africa's recent history which has already begun cannot form the basis of any realistic attempt to promote the necessary healing of this highly distorted health care system, I am inclined to echo what William L. Garrison wrote, back in 1831:

> I will be as harsh as truth, and as uncompromising as justice. On this subject, I do not wish to think, or speak, or write, with moderation. No! Tell a man whose

house is on fire, to give a moderate alarm; tell him to moderately rescue his wife from the hands of a rapist; tell the mother to gradually extract her baby from the fire into which it has fallen!—but urge me not to use moderation in a cause like the present.

References

1. World Health Organisation (WHO) (1983). *Apartheid and Health*. World Health Organisation, Geneva.
2. de Beer, C. (1984). *The South African Disease: Apartheid Health and Health Services*. South African Research Services, Johannesburg, South Africa.
3. West, M.E. and Boonzaier, E.A. (1989). Population groups, politics and medical science. *South African Medical Journal* **76**, 185–186.
4. de Beer, M., Padayachee, G.N., Ijsselmuiden, C., *et al.* (1993). The reliability of mortality data in Johannesburg. *South African Medical Journal* **83**, 597–601.
5. Phillips, H. (1990). The origin of the Public Health Act of 1919. *South African Medical Journal* **77**, 531–532.
6. Minter, W. (1986). *King Solomon's Mines Revisited: Western Interests and the Burdened History of Southern Africa*. Basic Books, New York.
7. ANC (1994). *A National Health Plan for South Africa*. African National Congress, Johannesburg, South Africa.
8. Bradshaw, D., Dorrington, R.E. and Sitas, F. (1992). The level of mortality in South Africa in 1985—what does it tell us about health? *South African Medical Journal* **82**, 237–240.
9. Slabber, C.F. (1992). A new South Africa—a new health care strategy. *South African Medical Journal* **82**, 388–391.
10. van Rensburg, H.C.J. and Fourie, A. (1994). Inequalities in South African health care. Part I: The problem—manifestations and origins. *South African Medical Journal* **84**, 95–99.
11. Zwarenstein, M.F. and Price, M.R. (1990). The 1983 distribution of hospitals and hospital beds in the RSA by area, race, ownership and type. *South African Medical Journal* **77**, 448–452.
12. Anon. (1972). *Report from South Africa*, South Africa House, London.
13. Simpson, M.A. (1988). Privatization: Boon or boondoggle? *Hospital Supplies*, Supplement: Private Health Care in South Africa, 38–41.
14. Simpson, M.A. (1988). *Privatization: Fantasy or Fact?* Plenary paper presented to the Conference: Spotlight on the Pharmaceutical Industry, Johannesburg, South Africa.
15. Simpson, M.A. (1988). The background to privatization: coping with the demand explosion. *Hospital Supplies*, Supplement: Private Health Care in South Africa, 86–89.
16. Simpson, M.A. (1990). Problems with privatisation. *South African Medical Journal* **78**(3), 168.
17. Broomberg, J., Chetty, K.S. and Masobe, P. (1992). The role of private hospitals in South Africa. Part I. Current trends. *South African Medical Journal* **82**, 329–334.
18. Kirsch, R.E. and Lee, N.C. (1992). A scalpel or an axe—should health cuts be brutalising or constructive? *South African Medical Journal* **82**, 298–299.
19. Lee, N.C. (1993). The public service labour relations shambles. *South African Medical Journal* **83**, 554.

20. Fabricus, H.J. (1993). The Public Service Labour Relations Bill of 1993—implications for the medical profession. *South African Medical Journal* **83**, 165–166.
21. Beattie, A., Doherty, J., Price, M., *et al.* (1992). Private practice in academic medicine—a Trojan horse. *South African Medical Journal* **82**, 385–386.
22. Hugo-Hamman, C.T., Vosloo, S.M., de Moor, M.M.A. and Odell, J.A. (1991). Paediatric heart transplants—should we do them? *South African Medical Journal* **80**, 434–436.
23. Lee, N.C. (1992). Transplants—who, what, where, when and how? *South African Medical Journal* **82**, 383.
24. Odell, J.A. and Brink, J.G. (1992). Heart transplantation in South Africa—a critical appraisal. *South African Medical Journal* **82**, 394–396.
25. Brink, J. and Pike, R. (1992). Transplantation in developing countries. *South African Medical Journal* **82**, 149–150.
26. Steyn, E. (1993). Towards a future policy for transplantation in South Africa. *South African Medical Journal* **83**, 712–713.
27. Myburgh, J.A. (1990). Surgery in South Africa: the interaction of specialization, the pursuit of excellence and the deployment of manpower. *Hospital Supplies* **16**, 18.
28. Benade, M.M. (1992). Distribution of health personnel in the Republic of South Africa with special reference to medical practitioners. *South African Medical Journal* **82**, 260–263.
29. Gear, H.S. (1937). A plea for improved South African medical and vital statistics. *South African Medical Journal* **11**, 149–154.
30. Botha, J.L. and Bradshaw, D. (1985). African vital statistics—a black hole? *South African Medical Journal* **67**, 977–981.
31. Davies, J.C.A. and Walker, A.R.P. (1990). We need more accurate data on the causes of sickness and death. *South African Medical Journal* **77**, 227–228.
32. Ncayiyana, D.J. (1994). Coming to grips with the future of health care—the ANC national health plan. *South African Medical Journal* **84**, 55–56.
33. Simpson, M.A. (1980). Epilogue: medical education and primary care. A critical review. In, *Medical Education and Primary Health Care*, ed. by H. Noack, Croom Helm, London.
34. Simpson, M.A. (1993). *Towards a New Health Care System for South Africa: obstacles and solutions.* Plenary paper presented to the Third Health Care Funding Conference, Midrand, South Africa, March 1993.
35. Simpson, M.A. (1993). Traumatic stress and the bruising of the soul: the effects of torture and coercive interrogation. In, *The International Handbook of Traumatic Stress Syndromes*, ed. by J.P. Wilson and B. Raphael, Plenum Press, New York.
36. PAC (1994). *The Transition Process, Reconstruction Programme, and New Health Planning for the Nation as Proposed by the Pan Africanist Congress of Azania*, Pan Africanist Congress, Johannesburg, South Africa.

Chapter 8

Health Care in Lithuania: From Idealism to Reality?

Eugenijus Gefenas

Institute of Philosophy, Sociology and Law, Vilnius, Lithuania

In this article I discuss 'the transition' of Lithuanian health care. In order to illustrate the size of the difficulties the people of Lithuania presently face, I focus in particular on the problem of resource allocation. I believe my observations (both general and particular) reflect the experiences of other post-socialist countries, especially those nations which were directly incorporated within the former USSR. Certainly, the two other Baltic states—Latvia and Estonia—have a great deal in common with Lithuania, both politically and culturally.

I have identified four questions to act as a framework for my discussion:

1. What were the main causes of the Soviet health care crisis?
2. What was the basis for resource allocation in the former socialist health care system?
3. What are the major obstacles set against the implementation of alternative principles of resource allocation in Lithuania?
4. What ideas might underlie and inform the design of a new Lithuanian health care system?

Resource Allocation within the Former Soviet Health Care System

The governing idea behind the distribution of health care resources in all socialist countries was the belief that diseases are the sign or product of an 'unjust' (or capitalist) society, and that only a 'just' (or communist) society is capable of eradicating disease: only communism possesses 'genuine concern and knowledge' about human needs and interests.

The general principle by which the distribution of medical goods and services was meant to be organised was—theoretically—*absolute egalitarianism*: 'for everyone according to his need'. The Soviet constitution explicitly entitled everybody to 'free and comprehensive medical care'. In addition to this general principle, it was said that health care policy should be based on a philosophy of prevention (at least this was the view of Semashco, the founder of the Soviet health care system).[1] Furthermore, in order to 'prevent disease' most efficiently, a strictly centralised, hierarchically managed health care institution was said to be required (this was referred to as a 'scientific' principle of management:[1] a similar idea was used in all spheres of Soviet society, in order to implement many other ideological claims).

The Lithuanian health care system was organised according to the same strict instructions which applied to all republics of the former USSR. The structure of individual health care institutions, the type and number of employees, and the supply of equipment, drugs and the like were all planned in Moscow. And, in practice, this meant that the abstract ideals of Soviet health care were never actually realised. The supposedly egalitarian distribution of medical resources was distorted by a two-tier system of health care institutions—the well-known 'special hospitals' offered a 'first-class' service to the Soviet 'nomenclature', while the rest of the population had access only to the far less well-resourced ordinary health care network. University clinics and central city hospitals formed part of the higher-tier health care system; and almost all the expensive, Western-made medical technology in the country was to be found at these elite clinics and hospitals. This obviously unequal distribution of resources was 'justified' by the assertion that this technology was necessary for scientific research (which was also said to be the best in the world).

Those who needed health care most of all—the mentally ill, the disabled and the handicapped—found themselves at the bottom of the health care pile. They were usually kept in 'special institutions' (not, of course, the first-class hospitals), or other places isolated from the 'egalitarian society'—and well away from the sight of foreigners.

Statistics which became available after the collapse of the old political system revealed that the grand claims made for the preventive power of the Soviet health care system were as fictitious as the 'egalitarianism'. It is now clear that mortality from conditions such as cardiovascular and repiratory diseases, cancers, accidents, and complications of pregnancy and childbirth had been increasing during the past few decades of socialist rule (as was the case throughout the former Soviet Union). In Lithuania today life expectancy for men is 67 years, and for women 76 years. In 1991 infant mortality was 14.7 per 1000 newborns, while the overall death rate has escalated over the past 30 years from 780 to 1060 per 100 000 population.

Stifling Authoritarianism

Despite the mythical nature of its main principles, the Soviet health care system did have an 'ethic' which was actually applied. Doctors swore to uphold 'communist morality' and 'the Soviet state' in the 'Oath of the Soviet Physician', and they did not have to take financial implications (for the system overall) into account while treating their patients. Personal autonomy was not regarded as important in the Soviet empire. As a result medical paternalism became an entrenched habit—indeed, the physician–patient relationship was just one aspect of the authoritarian and hierarchical spirit of all social relationships. The doctor was the expert on 'healthy life-style', and on medical technology and its application. From the ordinary patient's point of view, he was also a quite unchangeable element of a centralised, bureaucratic health care system.

The crisis of Soviet health care, and the failure of its preventive strategy was, to a large extent, caused by a stultifying mixture of paternalistic medical morality and Soviet ideology in general. The authoritarian ethos, and the total neglect of patient autonomy, ensured that health education appeared artificial, and was therefore ineffective. Furthermore, the denial that medical resources were scarce (how could they be under socialism?) actually heightened the inequalities of distribution across Soviet health care structures. Since there was no strain on health care resources, expensive medical units could be founded despite severe shortages. And, in establishing them, so the illusion of 'the best society', in which the most sophisticated modes of treatment were 'available for everyone . . .' was supposedly furthered.

The Lithuanian Economic Crisis, and its Influence on Health Care

In addition to those features of health care crisis which are common to all modern societies, some important differences characterise 'the transition period' of post-socialist health care. These are mostly to do with the imbalance between primary and specialised health care, and of course stem in the first place from an economic crisis which is especially deep in the countries of the former USSR.

Since 1990, Lithuanian economic output has declined by 50%, unemployment has reached 30%, and the rate of inflation rose to over 1000% in 1991–1992. Today, the average income of Lithuanians is one-third of what it was in 1991. This economic recession has had an enormous influence on health care financing. Ignoring conversion problems, and following the official exchange rate between the Lithuanian currency and the US$ (which is the most popular hard currency in our country), the Lithuanian health care budget amounts to approximately $50 million.[2] This means that annual health care expenditure is about $15 per person in Lithuania (Poland spends around $110, Britain $800, and the USA over $2500 per capita).[3] These figures cannot, of course, be directly compared because the prices of many goods are different in post-socialist and developed countries. At present, however, Lithuania is buying almost all medical equipment and drugs, as well as basic raw materials and energy resources, at world-wide prices.

The Situation Today: Disproportions, Rationing and Bribery

By far the most pressing problem facing the Lithuanian health care system is the aforementioned asymmetry between specialised and primary health care. This is a continuing legacy of the socialist system. In some university clinics and central hospitals physicians look after just three or four patients, and use very expensive medical equipment to do so, while there is a severe shortage of even the cheapest equipment in the countryside and in local hospitals.[2] Moreover, even though approximately 50% of infant mortality in Lithuania is due to poor prenatal care—and there is a widespread lack of appropriate technology and training to deal with the complications of labour[4]—units for low birth-weight babies nevertheless exist, and are in operation. We also possess high-tech clinics for heart surgery and organ transplantation. For example, in spite of severe economic crisis and a shortage of resources for primary care medicine (a lack of such basics as disposable syringes, antibiotics, vaccines, etc.) the seventh heart transplantation was performed in Lithuania in December 1993. The chief of Vilnius University clinic for heart surgery estimates the cost of this procedure to be about US$3000.[5]

According to the present-day Lithuanian Ministry of Health there is an over-supply of beds for surgery and child health care, on the one hand, and a shortage of beds for nursing and rehabilitation on the other. There are also disproportions between the number of medical personnel and medical equipment. For example, in 1991 there were more than 17 000 medical doctors (46 per 10 000 population) in Lithuania, twice as many doctors per person as in Western countries. At the same time, just to draw level with provision in the West, Lithuanian medical institutions would require 10 times more technical equipment.

The primary health care institutions (the so-called polyclinics) continue to function more as 'sick-list distributors' than useful sources of medical care. A combination of queuing, medical utilitarianism and bribery (an inevitable feature of all spheres of social life where queuing is necessary) has, for a long time, been the most common mode of rationing scarce biomedical resources. At present, the threat of unemployment has significantly reduced the queues in the polyclinics, and so too the waiting lists in local hospitals (sick people are less employable). However, retired people and indigent Lithuanians with very small incomes still try to get into hospital in order to improve their living conditions: a month's hospital food costs twice as much as the minimum monthly salary.[2]

Following the fairly recent inauguration of some private clinics and pharmacies in Lithuania, the ability to pay has—explicitly—been the new mode of rationing. However, in the forseeable future it is unlikely that more than a small percentage of our population will be able to afford to use the services. Bribery (a tacit form of the ability to pay) is even more prevalent than it used to be. Bribes help patients to 'jump the queue', to be admitted to a central hospital, or simply to be a little more confident about the quality of the medical service they will receive. Public resistance to 'tipping' is also on the wane these days, partly because a physician's salary amounts to only $20 per month (about 65% of the average Lithuanian salary).[2] Indeed, there are well-known 'tipping rates' for different biomedical services. For example, reimbursements for care during labour range from $20 to $50, dependent on the length and type of delivery:

> 'My ward neighbour gave $30. Therefore everything was OK. The midwife earned her two months salary during the night. It seems to be just, though. That hellish job is worth even more'—writes a woman in a newspaper called *Physician's News*.[6]

Overall, while simple queuing remains the popular official mode of rationing, other rationing criteria remain quite unexplicit. There have, for example, been no public discussions about the withdrawal of life-sustaining treatment, or of triage cases in Lithuania. It seems to be accepted that rationing decisions are simply part of the general process of medical decision-making.

Reorganising Health Care: The Enormous Task

In post-socialist Lithuania the majority of the population find it very difficult to obtain a decent minimum of health care. Undoubtedly, the whole structure of our health care institutions needs to be changed, and a new system created which will respond first to the most basic health care needs. If reasonable health care is to be provided for all Lithuanians, it seems particularly obvious that the expensive high-tech enclaves can no longer be allowed to continue at their previous level of activity.

However, two major obstacles stand in the way of a smooth transition to a new and fairer health care system. The first is the absence of primary care medicine (which might be understood as 'accessible, comprehensive, co-ordinated, and continual care given by accountable providers of health services').[7] The existing polyclinics have never provided such services. Indeed, the specialty of 'family doctor' has only recently been formally introduced in Lithuania. Thus, considerable time and resources are needed merely to create a rudimentary working structure of primary care medicine.

Secondly, the task of reorganising the specialised medical units is potentially even more difficult and painful, because the majority of skilled and experienced medical personnel stand to lose the opportunity to do their favourite jobs. The picture is further complicated by the fact that health care reform is being planned and will by implemented, by the medical elite. Very often, of course, these people have a personal interest in continuing their scientific research and sophisticated medical activities (which are, as a rule, impossible without modern technology).

The Lithuanian 'National Conception of Health': A Self-imposed Conceptual Challenge

In addition to the obvious practical barriers: the economic crisis, the severe shortage of health care resources, and the generally irrational structure of health care, a sensible programme of health care reform is up against some tough conceptual obstacles.

The official reform plan—the 'Lithuanian National Conception of Health'—emphasises the need to reorganise the system so as to prioritise preventive and primary health care. However, the plan has not been thought out, but is based on utopian ideas. The new 'conception of health' (which is modelled on the World Health Organisation's notion of targets for 'Health for All') declares that 40% of health problems are the result of human life-style, 30% are caused by environmental factors, 20% depend on genetics, and 10% are directly influenced by medical institutions. It is also claimed that 80–90% of health problems can be solved by the effective functioning of primary care medicine, and that this is the way to save resources for specialised medical care which ought to be provided in university centres.[8] However, as is the case with many WHO declarations, the terminology is very vague. The phrase 'primary care medicine' seems to be used to include such measures as preventive medicine, emergency medicine, health education and environmental control—but this is surely to over-emphasise the importance of medical work. However, leaving aside the lack of conceptual clarity, can even the basic premises be said to be correct?

Those who are sceptical about preventive medicine claim that it is extremely difficult to change people's life-style, and of course there is a well-known range of moral controversy associated with health education which cannot be avoided.[9,10] What is much more clear is that mortality and morbidity figures—and the effectiveness of health education—are strongly linked to the general economic situation.[11] The successful prevention of disease is very often a by-product of such general social progress as ending poverty, eliminating unemployment, ameliorating housing, and better general education for the population as a whole.

The idea that scarce health care resources can be saved through the implementation of preventive measures is also highly questionable. Preventive medicine extends human life and improves its quality, but at the same time it merely postpones the need for expensive curative medicine.[12]

To prioritise preventive medicine seems to be a cheap and attractive option to many countries trying to reorganise their health care, especially so to those who are doing so in deep economic crisis. However, the experience of other developed countries, as far as we can judge in our relative academic isolation, shows that the situation is vastly more complicated than it presently appears to our planners. To be able to reform Lithuanian health care intelligently we must first of all be realistic.

References

1. Semaschco, N.A. (1922). *Science on the Health of Society*. (Social Hygiene). (In Russian).
2. Cerniauskas, G. (1993). *Financing Health Care in Lithuania*, Report of the Lithuanian Ministry of Health. (In Lithuanian).

3. Blank, R.H. (1992). Setting policy priorities for allocating scarce medical resources. In, *Emerging Issues in Biomedical Policy, Vol. 1*, ed. by R.H. Blank and A.L. Bonnicksen, Columbia University Press, New York.
4. Ministry of Health (1993). *The Main Problems of the Lithuanian Health Sector in the Transition Period*. Report of the Lithuanian Ministry of Health.
5. Liutkeviciute, I. (1993). The heart and the kidneys of young suicide were transplanted to three patients. *Lithuanian Morning* **252**, 2. (In Lithuanian).
6. Radzeviciene L. (1993). The husband was together. *Physician's News* **27**, 91. (In Lithuanian).
7. Smith, H.L. and Churchill, L.R. (1986). *Professional Ethics and Primary Care Medicine*, Duke University Press, Durham.
8. *Lithuania MCMXC: Health and its Problems*. (1993). Medicina, Kaunas. (In Lithuanian).
9. Moskop, J.C. (1992). Confronting health care rationing. In, *Emerging Issues in Biomedical Policy, Vol. 1* ed. by L.H. Blank and A.L. Bonnicksen, Columbia University Press, New York.
10. Dougherty, C. (1993). Bad faith and victim-blaming: the limits of health promotion. *Health Care Analysis* **1**(2), 111–119.
11. Majnoni d'Intignano, B. (1993). *Financing Health Care in Europe*. Lietuvos SAM, Vilnius. (In Lithuanian, original French).
12. Hackler, C. (1993). Health care reform in the United States. *Health Care Analysis* **1**(1), 5–13.

Part Two:
Beneath the Cracks—Health Reform and Social Justice

Chapter 9

Going off the Dole: A Prudential and Ethical Critique of the 'Healthfare' State

Stuart F. Spicker

Center for Ethics, Medicine and Public Issues, Baylor College of Medicine, Houston; Emeritus Professor, University of Connecticut School of Medicine, USA

Part I: Introduction: From the 'Haves' to the 'Have nots'

When people have no insurance cover to reimburse health care providers and hospitals for health care costs incurred, and cannot afford to pay for health care themselves, the inevitable occurs: health care often becomes charity doled out not only by philanthropic institutions, primarily hospitals, but also by physicians and other health care providers who, from the virtue of charity, are moved to do so; but of course not all half million physicians in the US are so moved. Indeed, on 31 January 1989, Lawrence K. Altman, in his column in the *New York Times* was given the headline: 'Doctors are urged to donate more medical care to the poor'. The physician/reporter opened with the following remark: 'Medical leaders are urging doctors to renew their ancient traditions and donate more care to the poor'.[1] Dr Altman points out that physicians with prestige, like James E. Davis, President of the American Medical Association, recently claimed that 'taxpayer subsidies of [physicians'] education have added to a basic responsibility to see that they take care of the poor and needy of their community'. Behind such remarks is the tacit judgement that physicians today are more stingy and self-interested than their brethren of the past. But even if it is not true that many physicians are stingy in donating to charities and to individually sick patients, is it not a mere presumption (if not sheer folly) to

Reforming Health Care: The Philosophy and Practice of International Health Reform.
Edited by D. Seedhouse. © 1995 John Wiley & Sons Ltd.

believe that doling out health care in 'a patchwork of charity care'[2] could really alleviate the current crisis with respect to the plight of some 32–35 million medically uninsured people in the US? Clearly Dr Altman is correct when he says that '... because the number of uninsured people who need medical care far exceeds the philanthropic potential of health professionals and institutions, few would expect the medical profession to solve the problem itself'.[1] And even if more physicians wanted to offer charity and provide 'free' care to the indigent, our nation's complex health care provider models—health maintenance organisations (HMO), preferred provider organisations (PPO), and other medical corporations—make it virtually impossible to do so, because within such contexts decisions regarding the doling out of care in the form of charity would in all likelihood be made by the administrators and managers of these models whose very jobs depend on sticking to budgets and remaining in the black. Moreover, though many hospitals provide extensive charity care, many provide very little and some none at all, and self-employed physicians who admit patients to these institutions may have great difficulty doling out free care since there are additional and powerful disincentives for not doing so, namely:

1. Hospital administrators do not want their institutions to provide free health care that will exacerbate the present financial burden.
2. Physicians usually anticipate being reimbursed for their services.
3. These same physicians do not wish to take the risk of practising medicine without malpractice insurance coverage, which, however, is only one expensive item among others.

How are these and other costs to be borne when no remuneration is forthcoming from charitable care—aside from federally supported programmes such as Medicaid and Medicare? Put in simplest terms, we are constantly reminded that the indigent *need* housing, food, some cash, and numerous other things out-of-pocket cash can purchase, among which is access to health care providers and institutions, and subsequently medication, surgery, hospital admission, and long-term care. These overwhelming needs, and other factors as well, have led the US as well as a number of European nations to adopt a *welfare* ('healthfare') state. Welfare-state societies have frequently generated a dismal state of affairs, and it is now clear to most that generally speaking welfare and healthfare programmes have failed, continue to fail, and unless we soon extricate ourselves from this financing model, we may well find ourselves in even greater financial distress. From the standpoint of those in the US who influence health care economics, generally speaking they are not willing to permit the real gross national product (GNP) for health care to increase much beyond its current $14.0 + \%$;[3,4] the recent movement federally to regulate the nation's health care expenditures is testimony to this new policy.

The core of the problem created by welfare and healthfare is not only the 'flexible' if not simply inconsistent way the principle of welfare is applied—e.g. at times the assets of the haves are transferred to the have nots on the basis of *age*, at other times on the basis of *location*, at still other times on the basis of *merit*, yet quite often on the basis of *need*—but the fact that nothing from the recipient is required in return for being on the dole: there's no reciprocity for living off the dole. But *reciprocity* is (as we shall soon argue) morally relevant to a democratic polity. The current 'system' of providing welfare to those in need and even those who simply legitimise the system—the deserving poor[5]—simply continues to perpetuate itself, with little if anything in return to the indigent in the long run. Paradoxically, the standard interpretation of the purposes of welfare programmes, in which the haves or non-poor are *not* meant to benefit, has recently been challenged: that is, the non-poor can actually be shown to benefit significantly in a welfare-state society, and the distress among the poorer elements of society is therefore *not* relieved at the expense of the better off members. If this thesis is correct, as Goodin, Le Grand, and others have argued[6] then the defenders of the modern healthfare state are not only on weak ground *conceptually* (as I shall argue), but they are *empirically* mistaken in their understanding of the actual outcomes of welfare-state societies, like the current industrialised countries of Western Europe and North America: the relief of the needy and distressed by the less distressed becomes exposed as the political and ethical myth it is.[7,8]

Although the process of welfare-state formation began at different times, proceeded at different rates, and took different forms in European and North American countries, these welfare systems and 'social policies' share some characteristic features that transcend these differences: they are notorious for failing not in compassion but in not preparing for *unintended outcomes*, like minimising free choice and by creating disincentives to those able-bodied and capable of work; hence individuals are simply encouraged to elect to remain unemployed. The despairing outcome of the failure to utilise self-interest and resourceful and benign motivation so crucial to individual production and achievements of all sorts—absent force—has been known for centuries, one of the most well-known expressions being found in Adam Smith's *An Inquiry into the Nature and Causes of the Wealth of Nations*, where in one passage Smith digresses while describing the investment of capital and 'the invisible hand' that promotes ends particular individuals do not intend. He writes:

> By pursuing his own interests [the individual] frequently promotes that of the society more effectually than when he really intends to promote it. I have never known much good done by those who affected to trade for public good. It is an affectation, indeed, not very common among merchants, and very few words need be employed in dissuading them from it.[9]

In Chapter 5 of the same classic in political economy ('no longer required reading', Ginzberg[3] regrets, 'much less study, for the current generation of doctoral students in economics'), Smith remarks:

> The natural effort of every individual to better his own condition, when suffered to exert itself with freedom and security, is so powerful a principle, that it is alone, and without any assistance, not only capable of carrying on the society to wealth and prosperity, but of surmounting a hundred impertinent obstructions with which the follies of human laws too often incumber its operations; though the effect of these obstructions is always more or less either to encroach upon its freedom, or diminish its security.[9]

Smith's confidence in the principle that there is a 'natural effort of every individual to better his own condition' through employment and work was, however, a qualified confidence; for he also intended to establish rules to govern the market-place. The state must first provide *security* in order that each individual may remain *free* to better his own condition, and thus every individual must be permitted to remain generally unregulated and unconstrained by laws that tend to obstruct him as he proceeds to 'exert' himself. The commitment to each individual's freedom clearly runs counter to and conflicts with a government's decision to exercise its power and tax its citizens without *legitimate moral authority*. Legitimate authority may indeed exist, but it ought to be morally *legitimated*. That is, governments at times are required to account for their exercise of revenue collection, and my argument thus far is that welfare-state governments have proffered no convincing *moral* arguments to justify transferring the assets of the haves to the have nots in order, for example, to provide healthfare to the poor. That is, at the very least some *moral* argument is required to justify a government's exercise of its legal action with respect to the haves, while at the same time avoiding anarchism. Of course, governments *claim* legal authority to tax their citizens; if pressed for the source of moral authority, the overriding of the freedom of individuals has been 'justified' on the grounds of (1) *compassion*, (2) *duty* of government to its citizens' well-being (health being?), on the basis of having received, albeit tacitly, 'the consent of the governed' (a spurious claim, indeed), and on the basis of straightforward *prudential grounds*, in contrast to moral grounds, i.e. the pragmatic benefit of maintaining a large and healthy working force as well as a militia to maintain national security.

Part II: The Need for Health Care and Health Insurance

An appeal to the language and discourse of needs of the deserving poor in the US or to the principle of solidarity in some European nations, is to my mind simply inadequate. Let me illustrate by turning to so-called 'needs claims'.

First, there is usually no great problem when we consider general needs such as housing, food, and health care. We can usually agree that the 'homeless' require or need some form of shelter in order to live; similarly, the indigent need access to health care—whether 'minimum' or 'maximum' I shall not consider here[10]—in order to recuperate and often to remain well. Most people believe that governments, as guarantors of life and security, have a responsibility to provide for the need for health care. However, like Plotinus, as soon as we descend from this supreme and 'perfect' ideal need, we are immersed in controversy. What, more concretely, do those without private resources or health insurance *need* in order to be secured in health? What specific forms should the provision of health care take once we acknowledge the general need for health care? Do those without access to health care need forbearance to enter any hospital's emergency room for a short visit when symptoms or signs of illness appear? Do they need an acute care bed for a week or 10 days, an intensive care bed for a month, a long-term care bed for a year or more? Suppose the last, what kind of long-term care or chronic care institution is needed? As one recuperates, is he or she to receive subsidised housing to fulfil the need? Is the housing to be conveniently located near a shopping centre or easily accessible by public transportation or wheelchair-access vehicles? What else is needed to avoid the need for readmission to the hospital? Does he or she need health care subsidies, income support, a job, job training, or education? Do we really need to reformulate national health care policy such that, for example, tax incentives would be made available to encourage private investment in health care institutions? Perhaps we need to institutue further cost controls on health care—the very thing that might have made possible the purchase of health care for many of the employed who never had and still do not have health insurance, or who had but no longer have health insurance? Is furthering the healthfare state the solution if we truly value our freedom and the freedom of others—for many of today's have nots may well be tomorrow's haves? Let us be more specific and review the latest health care insurance situation in the US.

Seven years ago, an important but virtually unknown analysis of the dynamics of health insurance loss by those previously possessing such insurance (excluding for the moment those 10s of millions who never had, nor have ever acquired through employment, such insurance coverage) was conducted by staff economists, Alan C. Monheit and Claudia L. Schur, at the National Center for Health Services Research and Health Care Technology Assessment (NCHSR).[11] This study—the first to analyse health insurance status in detail in the US over time—covers the *transition* between having and not having health insurance. One of the results of this study is that approximately 8.4 million of the 242 million US residents—a quarter of the nation's 30–33 million [estimates are as high as 37 million][12] health uninsured—had neither private insurance nor public coverage for health care needs during a period of nearly three years.[11] Moreover, it was determined that public coverage was found to play a very small role in protecting persons from losing private coverage, and dependents were proportionally bigger losers of coverage than the primary insured. 'Of all those who lost coverage, 63% had dependent coverage, whereas only 53% of all the privately insured were dependents'.[11] Hence, young people (who as a group are typically much healthier than older people) still bear much of the burden: 'among persons who have lost private coverage, more than a third are children 18 years or younger and more than half are less than 25 years of age'.[11] Most importantly, however, the researchers determined that the 'long-term unin-sureds, compared with all persons who lose coverage, are a much more economically disadvantaged group with far less labour market attachment and less access to employment-related insurance',[11] thus tying the lack and loss of health insurance *primarily* to employment, that is *unemployment* itself (though, we should note, employers running small business do not, indeed, often cannot, offer health insurance to their employees). As a result, in addition to payments by the haves (the patients), in the US the employer and the taxpayer *combined* pay for or *subsidise by healthfare* a $550 billion ($0.5 trillion in 1987) annual health care bill for just about everyone.[4] Instead of advocating a policy and strategies that would encourage employment, and instead of confronting the political and moral premises of their proposed solutions, the authors of the study advocate a 'range of policy responses', among which are the usual tax credits and increased subsidisation that enable the able-bodied unemployed to share in paying the premiums 'between the former employer' and themselves as enrolees 'to reduce the out-of-pocket premium costs to the latter'.[11] But the existence of 'workers' presumes employers, not 'former employers', so that workers themselves can pay the bulk of the cost of their premiums for health insurance. Surely, we should welcome proposals that would 'contribute to a reduction in the size of the [health] uninsured population',[11] but perhaps not at any price, especially not at the price of incrementally decreasing the number of haves while increasing the numbers of those who will live off the dole. In short, it is difficult to agree with these economists when they say that it 'may be best [to expand] public insurance coverage, especially through the Medicaid programme' or a federally run uniform system of health insurance coverage, as ways of addressing the plight of the long-term or 'chronically uninsured'.[11,13,14]

Healthfare—The Moral Dilemma

The critical dilemma in the struggle to solve the problem of the health care needs of the poor, then, is as follows:

Premise 1. If (paraphrasing Samuel Johnson) a society lets its people remain destitute, starve in the streets, and go without a 'decent provision' of health care, then it *fails to be civilised and compassionate*; and, if a society advocates and carries out welfare policies rooted in fulfilling the needs of the have nots by transferring the assets of the haves to them without the haves' formal consent or moral authority (where continued reliance on the customary *assumption* of consent in a representative democracy is challenged), then that society *violates the moral rule of respecting the freedom of individuals* and this is unjustified (i.e. immoral).

Premise 2. Either a society does not provide a basic standard or 'adequate minimum' of health care to the have nots (whose personal worth we may assume is at least equal to the worth of the haves), or it adopts and carries out a healthfare policy that is designed to do so.

Conclusion. Such a society is either uncivilised and lacking in compassion, or it fails to respect the stern but minimum demands of morality.

Part III: Escaping between the Horns of the Dilemma

Like the 'horny' problem it is, the negative alternatives that constitute the conclusion of this complex argument need not be accepted without challenge. We can and should challenge the truth of the premises, or at least one of them. If successful, of course, the argument remains valid, but the conclusion will have been refuted, and we shall escape being 'impaled' by either of the 'horns' of the dilemma. That is, we may be able to proffer an argument that does *not* require the conclusion either that we shall become (1) a brutal and uncompassionate society, or (2) a society that sings the praises of its citizens' freedom while at the same time violating that freedom by unjustifiably transferring the assets of the haves to the have nots via significant taxation without the formal consent of the haves. Consider the disjunctive second premise: Is it not false? To be sure, we can imagine non-welfare (non-healthfare) societies that do enable all their citizens to have access to a range of health care options, i.e. from minimum to maximum, perhaps multi-tiered access and care levels. Furthermore, we can imagine non-healthfare states in which governments do not set out to restrict the freedom of purchase of very expensive treatments by the haves—e.g. organ transplants, the use of imaging technologies, long-term adjuvant therapies, and long-term care—primarily because these care options are left to the open market economy and may well become affordable by means of private insurance and out-of-pocket payments. In short, strict healthfare programmes are not the only options available in the US. We can conceivably make the transition to another set of social policy strategies. Perhaps we in the US must do so soon. But first we are obliged to demonstrate the *unethical* nature of welfare and healthfare.

Part IV: Transition to the Ethical Critique of the Healthfare State

At this point let me be perfectly clear: first, I am not arguing that health care should not be financed by private insurance, but only that it should not be financed by *government-run* insurance programmes (though government can provide the 'enabling conditions' which include protecting the market economy), since the revenues required would be (as they are now) unduly exacted from the nation's citizens. Indeed, I believe the US is now able to begin to move properly toward adopting a health care financing plan that will be tightly connected to a private insurance model, where individual citizens remain free not only to self-actualise through productive employment but also to determine the level of health care they prefer as well as the premiums they desire and elect to purchase from private firms.

In two January 1989 issues of the *New England Journal of Medicine*, Alain Enthoven and Richard Kronick (of the Graduate School of Business at Stanford University), offered a plan which would achieve nearly universal health care insurance coverage by permitting 'a diversity of health plans (non-profit and for profit) in the private sector such as now exists in the US'.[15] Happily, the plan is based on consumer choice, and not on government as the source of payment. These planners appreciate the fact that US citizens no longer have any taste for income redistribution, and they believe their plan 'does not have to involve extensive redistribution'.[15] Notwithstanding their general disclaimer, however, they write:

> Inevitably, in the case of the poorest people, who cannot be expected to pay the cost of their care, others with higher incomes must help them, just as they do today. But our proposal would raise a large part of the needed funds from non-poor working people who are uninsured today.

Finally, they hope 'if taxpayers of more ample means were willing to take on the burden of covering the poor, we would consider it to be all to the good'. The final irony, given the failure, both empirical and conceptual of the healthfare state, is captured in their remark: 'But it is important for low-income people to have health care coverage, even if they must pay a substantial part of the cost themselves'.[15]

Clearly, Enthoven and Kronick are unwilling to project a plan that will take citizens off the dole, although they seem deeply committed to a strategy of 'managed competition' that ought not to be put in place too quickly and that must avoid 'radical discontinuity with the present'. But their proposal, like so many others before them, does not attack the heart of the problem—the massive numbers of unskilled, uneducated, illiterate and unemployed we call our neighbours. Until this situation is attacked by massive education and training programmes, only patchwork remedies will remain.

Second, by now it should be obvious that I am not defending further tampering with current payment systems that in the end only shuffle the costs and expenditures around—from cheques the haves currently send to insurance companies to cheques they would henceforth send to the US Internal Revenue Service (IRS). Indeed, here I call for a non-welfare, non-healthfare model, in which it will be necessary for the haves to send cheques in precisely the other direction: not to the IRS but to various insurance firms (though federally and state regulated) in the private sector, leaving an additional amount to be sent to the IRS earmarked for investment in a wide variety of nationally subsidised education and training programmes that in the end are directed to the well-being of all affected individuals.[16] This approach, designed to enable the have nots to become the moral agents for their economic choices, though admittedly involving a complex plan, requires that the US government and the 50 states collect and transfer significant revenues, directing them in the form of *investment* in nationally-supported educational and training programmes for eligible citizens, since there is some evidence that this is the most likely way the US can significantly reduce its unemployment.[7,8] For in today's US healthfare state, only one in 25 trainees actually finds a job. However, if we begin now and proceed *gradually*, over a period of 15–20 years we can remove the current welfare and healthfare recipients 'away from the dole and toward escape from the dole . . .'.[7,17] The evidence is surely mounting to suggest that US citizens are no longer willing to pay the costs of financing their current healthfare non-system; moreover, we in the US have learned that in perpetuating the present system we unjustifiably continue to interfere with our citizens' freedom by taking resources from the haves and transferring them to the have nots without reciprocity and, paradoxically, without much in the way of long-term benefit to the have nots. We must begin to rein in what has run amok.

The need to initiate nationwide educational and training programmes that *invest* tax revenues toward and *temporarily subsidise* each citizens' education (e.g. eliminating illiteracy) and training (e.g. the unskilled mastering one or more skills), places *rationality and social intelligence* at least on a par with *individual freedom*. This, I now hope to show, is in sharp contrast to the present healthfare state, which, in interfering with the individual freedom of the haves, by-passes the opportunity for sound investment in the have nots, and thus discourages the future possibility of reciprocity by those recipients on the dole. In short, my thesis includes the claim that *individual freedom is not, as uncompromising libertarians would have it, an absolute side constraint*; indeed, individual freedom may be legitimately restricted by state and federal authorities but only in the name and act of encouraging, producing, sustaining, and reinforcing the ends of *rationality and social intelligence*. The theory and policy I advocate and have sought to defend here, then, is therefore neither inherently emancipating nor inherently repressive, calls for democratic and egalitarian social change, and belongs properly under the rubric of a more compromising, that is, 'quasi' libertarianism.

Part V: Values in Tension: Individual Freedom vs Social Intelligence

The radical libertarian view, we are reminded, takes each individual's freedom as a 'side constraint'. That is, the value status of a person is such that he or she is to remain uncoerced and respected (*pace* the freedom of others in reciprocity) as the fundamental source of self-imposed law, i.e. as autonomous. (Here we need not trace the fact that the individuality or personhood of human beings had to be created as much as discovered; suffice to say the custom is now taken for granted in civilised states.) Singular persons, so to speak, are now emancipated and even expected to participate in the free play of initiative and various kinds of commercial activity. Throughout the process of and struggle for emancipation, the acquired and created liberty of the individual at one and the same time led to the condemnation of various social policies, i.e. welfare—for it denied in principle the voluntary choice of the haves, and it did not judge the authority of individual volition a sufficient force to shape social policies. Moreover, in ideal democratic polities one essential constituent is that each individual acquires the intelligence needed, under the operation of self-interest, to engage in the market-place and in political affairs. This is what Walter Lippmann once called the 'omnicompetent individual', educated and competent to exert himself or herself in the market-place as well as competent to frame policies, to judge their results, and be able to recognise those situations requiring political action aimed at his or her own good.[18] All this the welfare state inhibits. The knowledge or rationality of which I speak is neither modelled on nor to be confused with Platonic ideals, i.e. knowledge of concepts, but rather the knowledge and behaviour that results from human association, peer exchange, and especially the master/apprentice relationship. It is a knowledge that depends upon tools, e.g. computers, and what can and must be socially transmitted; in short, knowledge acquired through the transmission of social institutions.

Thus, we in the US must direct our energies and dollars toward the ends of achieving universal social intelligence and reasonableness in negotiation; only then will follow the possibility of universal health insurance.

Conclusion

At this point I am committed openly to acknowledge and advocate coercion via education to produce a society that can and must think and reason freely. This leads to a paradox: in stressing the value of individual liberty, I advocate coercing individuals to be trained or even to master what is entailed by the goals of social intelligence and reasonableness in negotiation. Educators, of course, have always understood this paradox; they have often justified coercing the young to learn, and have always defended the need to do so. While valuing 'freedom to' (in contrast to 'freedom from') as highly as we do and should, we also appreciate the fact that freedom encounters a challenger of equal stature—the goal of each citizen's rational self-sufficiency.

The motto of Sweden's Uppsala University, which I noticed when visiting some years ago, comes to mind: 'Tänka Fritt Är Stort men tänka ratt Är Större' ('To think free is great, but to think right is greater still'). This is a far cry from the maxim of the healthfare state: To eat right is great, but to eat free is greater still.

References

1. Altman, L.K. (1989). Doctors are urged to donate more medical care to the poor. *New York Times* (January 31):B-7.
2. Tallon, J.R. (1989). A health policy agenda proposal for including the poor. *Journal of the American Medical Association* **261**, 1044.
3. Ginzberg, E. (1992). Health care and the market economy—a conflict of interest? *New England Journal of Medicine* **326**(1), 72–74.
4. Enthoven, A. and Kronick, R. (1989). A consumer-choice health plan for the 1990s: universal health insurance in a system designed to promote quality and economy. (Part 1) *New England Journal of Medicine* **320**, 29–37; (Part 2) **320**, 94–101.
5. Halper, T. (1973). The new 'deserving poor' and the old. *Polity* **6**, 71–86.
6. Goodin, R.E. and Le Grand, J. (1987). *Not Only the Poor: The Middle Class and the Welfare State*, Allen & Unwin, London.
7. Murray, C.A. (1984). *Losing Ground: American Social Policy, 1950–1980*, Basic Books, New York.
8. Murray, C.A. (1988). *In Pursuit of Happiness and Good Government*, Simon and Schuster, New York.
9. Smith, A. (1776). *An Inquiry into The Nature and Causes of The Wealth of Nations*, ed. by E. Cannan (1965), Modern Library, New York.
10. Abel-Smith, B. (1978). Minimum adequate levels of personal health care: history and justification. *Milbank Quarterly* **56**, 7–21.
11. Monheit, A.C. and Schur, C.L. (1988). The dynamics of health insurance loss: a tale of two cohorts. *Inquiry* **25**, 315–327.
12. Thorpe, K.E., Siegel, J.E. and Dailey, T. (1989). Including the poor: the fiscal impacts of Medicaid expansion. *Journal of the American Medical Association* **261**, 1003–1007.
13. Himmelstein, D.U. and Woolhandler, S. (1989). A national health program for the United States: a physician's proposal. *New England Journal of Medicine* **320**:102–108.

14. Relman, A.S. (1989). Universal health insurance: its time has come. *New England Journal of Medicine* **320**, 117–118.
15. Enthoven, A. and Kronick, R. (1989). A consumer-choice health plan for the 1990s: universal health insurance in a system designed to promote quality and economy. (Part 2) *New England Journal of Medicine* **320**, 94–101.
16. Moffit, R.C. (1992). Surprise! a government health plan that works. *Wall Street Journal* (2 April). Reprinted in the *Congressional Record—Extension of Remarks* (28 April 1992), E1101–1102.
17. Sampford, C.J.G. and Gilligan, D.J. (eds.) (1986). *Law, Rights and the Welfare State*, Croom Helm, London.
18. Zeidner, R. (1992). Choice in health benefits: too much of a good thing. *Government Executive* (April). Reprinted in the *Congressional Record—Extension of Remarks* (28 April 1992), E1102.

Editor's Note

This paper is the original version of a manuscript which was edited and shortened for inclusion in *Health Care Analysis*. The author requested that the full version be included in *Reforming Health Care*. Since his chapter is criticised in the following chapter of this collection Professor Spicker naturally felt that his views should be explained as comprehensively as possible. Dr Loughlin's critical analysis of Professor Spicker's paper is the version which appeared in *Health Care Analysis*.

Readers will quickly appreciate that the Spicker/Loughlin debate is emotionally charged. There is a lot at stake here, and each author knows this very well. Health reform may provide the specific focus for their discussion, but underneath their dispute is about the fundamentals of political philosophy.

Chapter 10

Health Reform and the Utopian Ideology of the New Right

Michael Loughlin

Manchester Metropolitan University, Crewe and Alsager College, Alsager, Cheshire, UK

Professor Spicker claims that the welfare state is both 'empirically' and 'conceptually' flawed. It seems that these claims correspond respectively to his 'prudential' and 'moral' critiques, but he does not make this link explicit, nor does he make clear what he means by these terms.

What might he mean? In Kantian philosophy the distinction between prudential and moral reasoning is made as follows: prudential reasoning proceeds from the assumption that one has certain goals, and concerns how one achieves them, while moral reasoning concerns what goals one should have in the first place. These types of reasoning are distinguished by their methods: while the former concerns matters of fact, being a search for the most efficient means to a given end, the latter is an *a priori* inquiry. Its methods concern the examination of key *concepts*, such as duty, the good, autonomy and choice, in order to discover what relationships they have with one another and with the concept of morality itself. This would explain why the author at one point describes his prudential critique as 'pragmatic', and why he seems to think that a moral critique of something shows that thing to be *conceptually* flawed.

The 'Prudential Critique'

I take Spicker's prudential critique to be the claim that, even if one happens to have the goal of helping the needy, the welfare state is not the way to do it.

Reforming Health Care: The Philosophy and Practice of International Health Reform.
Edited by D. Seedhouse. © 1995 John Wiley & Sons Ltd.

Specifically, if one wants to make people healthy, a system based on the principle of free access to health care for all who need it, paid for out of taxation, will not help to achieve this goal: in fact it will only exacerbate the problem.

Spicker's support for these claims is slight. He correctly points out that there are links between social deprivation and ill-health, such that providing medical services on the basis of need is *insufficient* to eliminate illness. But this shows that there are other things that have to be done *besides* providing free services to the needy: it does not necessarily and only follow that what has to be done must be done *instead* of providing such services.

Spicker's view is that there is something *in the nature* of welfare systems that makes them incapable of doing what they are meant to do, and that they actually contribute to the social problems they are designed to alleviate.

What defence is there of this view in the chapter? He writes:

> Welfare-state societies have frequently generated a dismal state of affairs, and it is now clear to most that generally speaking welfare and healthfare programmes have failed, and continue to fail.

But to whom does 'most' refer? By what standards are welfare-state societies deemed to have failed, and most seriously, what grounds does Spicker have for treating the existence of welfare programmes within the economies that have them as the cause of their failure? Certainly most people living in modern capitalist societies might agree that life is often far from perfect within such societies, and that the existence of poverty and preventable diseases in rich countries like the US is a remarkably 'dismal state of affairs'. However, out of the many political, social and economic forces at work in such countries, to identify one feature, the existence of welfare programmes, as 'generating' this state of affairs is to make a very strong claim. To substantiate it Spicker would need a lot of evidence: he would have to show, via a detailed sociological analysis of late 20th century Western societies, that without the existence of such programmes conditions would be better than they are now. Instead of such an analysis Spicker merely offers us some generalisations about 'human nature', backed up by a quotation by Adam Smith.

According to Spicker, the existence of welfare creates disincentives to work, such that 'individuals are simply encouraged to elect to remain unemployed'. It seems that the behaviour of 'the poor' (who can be understood as a largely homogeneous class) can be effectively analysed in terms of two simple dispositions, and it is these dispositions, not complex economic and political forces beyond their control, that constitute the cause of their poverty—in conjunction, of course, with the misguided actions of welfare-state liberals and lefties.

The poor (otherwise described by the ugly term 'the indigent') are lazy, so lazy that they would rather live on paltry benefits than work for a living. The folly of this choice is explained by the fact that they are also stupid: they are 'the unskilled, uneducated, illiterate unemployed we call our neighbours' (I notice we only *call* them our neighbours. I doubt that they are Spicker's neighbours in the physical sense of the word. Is this an allusion to the Good Samaritan parable and an answer to the question: 'Who is my neighbour'? The answer being, whoever doesn't *need* any help in the first place.)

Having diagnosed the problem, Spicker's solution follows swiftly. Obviously the illiterate, unskilled indigent need educating. They need to learn not only skills that make them useful to the market—they also need initiating into the ways of capitalist society, learning how to exercise something called 'economic and social rationality'. Only then can they 'become the moral agents of their own economic choices'.

The investment required for this education would be 'significant' but temporary—for if the state had to keep up this spending, generation after generation, then Spicker's proposal would be no advance on 'healthfare', since the burden of taxation would always remain. Spicker's faith in the free market to provide full employment, given only an educated labour force, is to say the least, optimistic: in which economic theories does he ground this claim? Even monetarists accept that in any advanced capitalist society there will be some unemployment.[1] Spicker seems to think that economics not only begins, but also ends with Adam Smith. He does not appear to have considered the claim that in a competition there must be losers as well as winners, nor has he thought what would happen if one of the newly educated ex-indigents was unpleasant enough to choose not to educate his or her own children. Would the state then step in, committing itself to ever-more public spending (for if I can get my child educated for free, wouldn't others soon learn about this and follow my lead?) or would that child live to spawn a new generation of illiterates? (Or is the reference to 'moral agents' meant to imply that the education Spicker has in mind would make us all excellent people, so that no one would ever make such a choice?) Furthermore, Spicker does not seem to have considered that not all poverty results from unemployment, but can equally be caused by *low pay*. In his Utopian world of skilled computer-operators and businessmen, who would do the jobs that those with such skills now pass up? Either the state would have to force employers to pay higher wages, violating *their* right to choose how to spend their own money and possibly causing them to get out of no-longer-profitable markets, or the state would have to subsidise services itself, which rather smacks of everything Spicker is trying to avoid.

The 'Ethical Critique'

So much for Spicker's prudential critique. What of his moral critique? The author has one fundamental moral premise: it is wrong to oblige some individuals to help others, without the consent of those so obliged, since to do so would be to violate their rights as autonomous beings. If true, this premise would rule out all redistributive policies as immoral, even those designed to supply such essential services as health care, since the taxation used to fund these policies is taken out of people's wages automatically, without obtaining their formal consent.

But the author supplies no argument whatsoever for his moral claim. Given that it is treated as a conceptual truth, he would need an *a priori* argument explaining the links between the concept of morality, rights and his specific concept of freedom. For it is not at all *obvious* that my freedom to refuse aid to those in more need than myself is a moral right, any more than it is obvious that my freedom to drive on the pavement is a moral right.

We do not think it is always illegitimate to limit freedom: you do not necessarily violate my rights by obliging me to do something which it is my duty to do anyway. Spicker would have to supply some argument to the effect that the needy have *no right* to our aid *before* claiming that obliging us to aid them violates our rights. He cannot just assume that this freedom to refuse aid is a moral right, and then conclude that the needy cannot have any rights against 'the haves'. To justify his views about which freedoms require respect, Spicker might appeal to the (somewhat dubious) distinction in right-wing moral philosophy between negative and positive liberty—were it not for the fact that he explicitly repudiates this distinction at the end of the article (saying we *rightly* value 'freedom to' as much as 'freedom from').

This point brings me to the chapter's most serious flaw. Supposing we accept Spicker's central moral claim, it immediately follows that his own proposal for a massive, state-funded education programme is as morally flawed as any of the welfare programmes he opposes. The fact that he claims (however implausibly) that the investment would only have to be temporary is quite beside the point. If taxation is the moral cousin of theft then continuous, systematic theft may be wrong, but short-term systematic theft is hardly legitimate.

Spicker's compromised, quasi-libertarianism is conceptually confused. The word 'compromise' doesn't function as a philosophical cure-all, and doctrines are not rendered consistent by placing the word 'quasi' in front of them. If the principle forbidding taxation is not an *a priori* moral truth, but can be compromised for utilitarian reasons, then the argument simply collapses. The more essential a service is, the more likely it is that we may be entitled to override the liberty of some to provide this service to others, and since health provision is the definitive essential service, it is legitimate to provide it to all who need it at the expense of those who can afford it, even when these two sets of people are not co-extensive.

As a final comment: ultimately the most revealing features of the chapter are its uses of language and inverted commas. Health care, which is provided or delivered to most of us, is *doled-out* to the *indigent*. Is Spicker implying that a different level of care or style of delivery is appropriate when dealing with non-paying patients? Or is the suggestion that health care professionals who work with the poor will naturally care less about what they do than those who work with the well-off?

Quotation marks can have many legitimate uses, but Spicker uses them throughout in the style of a popular journalist: to cast doubt on the legitimacy of a claim without any argument whatsoever. So we see that social policies he does not approve of are 'social policies', welfare-state systems are 'systems', and health care provided free to those who need it is provided 'free'. To take up only one of these uses: Spicker is presumably trying to draw our attention to the fact that allegedly free services are not really free, because they cost something to produce. But no-one who advocates free health care provision is denying this. The word 'free' does not mean *created ex nihilo*. Mail-order firms that offer 'free' gifts with your next purchase are not claiming to have miraculous powers. (Nor, in any other way, would they want to imply that the gift they are offering costs little or nothing to produce—quite the contrary.) They mean, simply, that the good offered will not cost anything to *the recipient*, over and above what has been paid already. So for free health care: you pay your contribution in taxes and no more, so that when you fall ill you will be provided for. Instead of pretending his opponents are committed to patently false empirical claims, Spicker should consider some of their moral arguments, such as socialist arguments for a link between the concepts of need and justice. Such arguments can be dismissed, however, because they are no longer to the 'taste' of 'US citizens' (another apparently homogeneous group).

But the most interesting use of quotes is Spicker's decision to place inverted commas around the word 'homeless'. He is *not* quoting anyone when he does this. The quotation marks therefore suggest that the homeless are not *really* homeless: they only say or think they are. This implication runs contrary to Spicker's acknowledgement that poverty does exist, and reveals something of his underlying attitude. He is in that tradition of American thinkers who believe that when social problems are discovered, it is usually our 'internal environment' that needs changing, not the 'external environment'. Autonomy is a state of mind, not subject to material constraints, which is presumably why we can make everyone autonomous just by 'educating' them (to use another Spickerism) into the ways of free-market capitalism. Once we change the way people think, the world will change: once we get the poor to stop thinking of themselves as poor and see that they are in fact potentially rich—once we get them to really 'go for it'—poverty will be eliminated. Utopian denial of the nature of reality, massive oversimplification of complex social relationships—these are the disturbing features of the ideology of the new right, and they are exemplified nowhere better than in Professor Spicker's chapter.

Reference

1. Friedman, M. (1968). The role of monetary policy. *The American Economic Review* **58**, 1–17.

Chapter 11

Of Markets, Technology, Patients and Profits

Erich H. Loewy

Department of Medicine, The University of Illinois College of Medicine, USA

Introduction

In the past few decades the costs of health care throughout the industrialised world have risen dramatically. Although the rates of such increase are quite different in different countries, the costs as well as the increase in such costs are greatest in the US.[1] Unless something definitive is done to halt or at least to moderate this rise, costs will predictably continue to escalate and threaten the quality of care as well as of research. The increase in costs can be attributed to many factors. Among these are:

1. The undoubted advances in the ability of medicine to diagnose and effectively treat illness, which has necessitated ever more technical skill on the part of physicians. This emphasis on technical skills has often led physicians to neglect other aspects of a case. Diagnosis or treatment merely because diagnosis or treatment is possible, and not because patients would really profit from such activities, often results in patients being kept alive beyond all reason to do so.
2. The rapid increase in the sophistication of diagnostic and therapeutic modalities, some of which may, for a variety of reasons, be inappropriately used: such reasons include, but are not limited to, fears of litigation, public demand and competition. This use of technology has, unfortunately, been at the expense of clinical skill and reasoning: instead of technology being used to supplement and assist reasoning, patients tend to be 'plugged into' technical devices.[2]

Reforming Health Care: The Philosophy and Practice of International Health Reform.
Edited by D. Seedhouse. © 1995 John Wiley & Sons Ltd.

Although basically the same technology exists in most parts of the industrialised world, there is a marked difference in the frequency with which such technology is used in various countries. Not surprisingly, and although by and large outcome statistics do not differ, the costs of the health care system in these various countries, measured by the proportion of the gross national product (GNP) used for health care differs markedly. Where outcome statistics differ, there is no correlation between 'the best' and 'the most expensive'.

In this chapter I explore the reasons for these differences. I focus on some of the conditions in the US, not only because I am both theoretically and practically familiar with them but especially because at least until now the health care system, as much else in the US, is and has been largely controlled by market forces. I argue against the theory that competition among health care providers and institutions, 'managed' or otherwise, can be relied upon to increase quality while decreasing costs.

Conditions Today

When one wishes to examine a society in which personal freedom is the predominant value, one can profitably turn to the US just as one can (or could have) profitably turned to the Soviet Union to examine a society in which personal freedom was sacrificed to the (at least theoretical) demands of the community. In both states the net result has been a large mass of unhappy, unfulfilled and often desperate people.

The health care system in the US (like much else in American society) tends to be bimodal: in places it is highly sophisticated and often truly superb; at others it is shoddy and inadequate. This health care system rides piggy-back on a society which, on the one hand, has unbelievable wealth (concentrated in the hands of a very few) and on the other poverty and squalor afflicting all too many.[3]

Social conditions in the US must be seen to be truly appreciated. Unfortunately middle- and upper-class Americans and their friends from other countries who visit them seldom see the situation. Many Americans are selectively blind: they simply fail to see what it is not convenient to see. Others are either so sheltered in their own environment that they fail to see what is almost next door or are, sometimes because of lack of imagination and sometimes because of amazing callousness, indifferent to it.

The Flesh and Blood of Poverty

The statistics I shall cite are well known but lack 'flesh and blood': they are not 'alive' as are real people and real situations. Therefore, I shall try to flesh them out by describing some real human situations. In the past few years the incidence of poverty and the numbers of the poor have become ever larger.[3-9] Not only does the traditional 'poverty class' (which is basically quite different in the US from some other Western nations: I shall have more to say about this later) continue to be poor; at a time when the wealthy have become ever more wealthy, more and more members of the lower-middle-class have lost their jobs and their possessions. At this time the 'upper' 1% of the population has more wealth and property than does the lower 90%.[9]

Partly because of pervasive poverty (as well as for a number of other reasons peculiar to American society) the streets of American cities (even of smaller cities) are quite dangerous: it is not rare that persons are attacked and injured at any time of the day or night. My wife was 'mugged' in front of the Watertower Complex in Chicago on a Tuesday afternoon, and a student of mine was raped on a weekday at about 7.00 pm on one of the larger streets of the small city in which I live. And often people are not only robbed but severely injured: slashing the face of the person who has just been robbed is a fairly common occurrence. Homelessness is widespread. Often the homeless are whole families with children; such homeless are quite visible in some of the parks surrounding the White House in Washington. Figures are hard to come by but it is estimated that there are between 1 and 2 million homeless. Hunger and malnutrition, in rural as well as in urban areas, is not unusual.[10] About one-third of children (and about one-half of black children) go to bed hungry: up from about one-fourth a few years ago.[10] Areas with stark poverty and hunger are often geographically not far removed from those in which the very wealthy spend huge sums for rent and eat only the most expensive foods. The amount spent on a day's luxuries by some of the wealthy often far exceeds the monthy income of a poor family.

Because of the way statistics are collected, it is not easy to be certain of the extent of unemployment. Statistics fail to count those who have been unemployed for more than a year or those who have given up seeking employment. People who have been unemployed for many years (and who not atypically come from families in which unemployment and hopelessness have become a 'tradition') will not appear in such statistics. Unemployment insurance (which varies between states) generally provides help for only 6 months: after that, unless the unemployed person is ill, or is the mother of dependent children, income stops. Such persons may then be eligible for welfare. Welfare in most states, however, is so constructed that it discourages people from seeking employment and encourages them to break up families: mothers who accept a low-paying job which carries no health insurance benefits and fails to provide day-care literally cannot afford to work and provide even minimally for their children and families. They are better off when the husband leaves than they are if they maintain the family unit (I know of fathers who on weekends secretly visit wives from whom they have officially separated!). In the black ghettos it is common for the majority (and at times almost all) to be unemployed or, if not, to earn too little to maintain even minimal standards.[11]

Being Poor, and Being in Poverty

It is important to differentiate between being poor and being in poverty. While many of us reading this book may have been poor (when I fled from Hitler I certainly was) I doubt that any of us has been in poverty. Being poor means going without adequate food or shelter, it may mean selling things on the street or even living, for a short time, on some form of the dole. But, because of a better yesterday and because of a tradition of success, those who are poor, as distinct from those who are in poverty, maintain the hope of a better tomorrow; in true poverty, even hope ceases to exist. A large number of America's people are not only poor; they are in poverty.

The upper and middle-middle-class in America live, at least materially speaking, extremely well. Members of the middle and lower-middle-class, however, live in constant danger: four weeks without a salary cheque would leave 60% of Americans bankrupt. Unfortunately, such people are often largely unaware of this looming reality and continue to oppose social programmes. Having been brought up as crass individualists they remain unconcerned until they are personally affected: and then it is too late!

People aged over 65 are generally entitled to social security payments: the amount of such payments hinges on previous earnings so that the very people who lack other pension plans or who, because of poor income, were unable to save are the very ones who receive least. As a result, a large number of the elderly, especially a large number of elderly women and Blacks, live in poverty.[12] It is little wonder that suicide among older people is far from rare, and has been increasing.

Bimodal Health Care

The health care system reflects the above circumstances: again, it is essentially bimodal. On the one hand, those who are better off are well insured and largely enjoy superb health care; those who are poor or poorly insured must do with sporadic and spotty charity.

The kind of insurance people have depends upon their employment. It is almost impossible to say just what is covered: each job carries a different kind of policy and such policies are apt to change over the years. Many cover most care quite generously; others are grossly inadequate; some pay only for inpatient but not for outpatient care or physician's fees. Most cover only a certain number of days in hospital: when illness is severe and when coverage is desperately needed, many policies will no longer cover. Illness can easily bankrupt a family.

People aged over 65 are entitled to Medicare. Medicare has two parts: the one is provided to virtually all over 65, the other must be bought by the insured. Part one, after patients have paid a 'deductible' themselves, covers hospital care. Hospital costs, however, are only for a certain number of days per year and nursing homes in general are not covered. Again, prolonged illness or severe debility can totally ruin a person: before being eligible for other help, people must have depleted all their funds so that savings, including the family home or care can easily disappear. Once the elderly have gone bankrupt, they become eligible for Medicaid. When patients have purchased 'part B' (which is not very expensive but may, despite this, be unaffordable for people living on minimal social security), they are entitled to outpatient care and laboratory and X-ray services. Medications and appliances, however, are not covered. Many of the elderly find it virtually impossible to buy medications or obtain appliances and are, therefore, in a position where they can obtain but not follow their physician's advice. My wife's aunt, who receives $370.00 in social security per month, for example, has a drug bill of about $200.00. A choice between eating and taking one's medication results: a choice which, since such patients are apt to become yet more ill, will drive up the ultimate costs of health care.

The 'really poor' are entitled to medical care; how being 'really poor' is defined differs from state to state. Medicaid pays for physician, hospital, laboratory, medications and nursing homes: but it pays providers so badly that they either refuse to accept such patients or are forced to practise an exceedingly inferior kind of medicine.

About 20% of Americans (and a larger percentage of children) lack insurance: they are neither poor enough to be on Medicaid nor have a job which provides insurance. These are not the unemployed but are usually people who have jobs which not only pay little but do not carry fringe benefits such as health insurance. They are, in terms of their medical care and often also otherwise, worse off than the unemployed; not entitled to Medicaid and not having insurance they fall between the two stools. One must add to this 20% another 25–30% of people who are severely underinsured.

Often people who are chronically ill or who, in the past, have had certain illnesses, find it impossible to get either insurance or a job: insurance companies may refuse to insure them and employers often are unable to hire them because their insurance carrier would raise premiums. Since insurance cannot be 'transferred' from one job to another, people may find themselves unable to quit their job: if they have had certain illnesses, the new carrier may not pick them up. Health care insurance thus often becomes the pivot about which everything else turns.

While there certainly is poverty in the rest of the industrialised world, it is generally a poverty of a different kind: not as stark, not as ingrained and traditional in many families, not as frequent and with better social supports. As far as health care is concerned, it is interesting that only South Africa and the US lack a health care system in which everyone is entitled to at least basic health care benefits.

Philosophy, World Views and the Market

The philosophy which underwrites the current state of affairs in the US, and indeed the philosophy on which capitalism is based, owes much to the rise of Protestantism as well as to the work of Thomas Hobbes and Adam Smith.[13-15] Protestantism with its emphasis on the individual, on individual choice and on individual salvation as well as tending to attribute material prosperity to personal merit (and, by default, poverty to personal failure) underwrote not only the rise of democracy (or rather its rediscovery since the idea of democracy is, of course, originally Greek) but also fostered the rise of capitalism.[13]

For Hobbes, the 'fundamental law of nature' is that a man should endeavour to bring about peace whenever there is any chance of it, and when there is no chance (as in 'the state of nature') then nothing morally prevents a man from taking all the necessary steps to protect himself. Hobbes' 'second law of nature' shows a path to peace. When each man lays down his right to self-protection he is 'contented with so much liberty against other men, as he would allow other men against himself'. However, such mutual trust is quite irrational in 'the state of nature': 'covenants, without the sword, are but words, and of no strength to secure a man at all'.[16] Thus Hobbes argued for an absolute monarchy. Impelled by mutual terror, self-interested people would agree to a social contract which, so long as they relinquished any claim to any other potential rights, would guarantee their protection by the sovereign. Hobbes' philosophy is based on fear and mistrust. There is no place in it for mutual aid—the idea that people might actually help each other is alien to his stark individualism.

Later philosophers, notably Nozick in general and Engelhardt in medical ethics, have made use of Hobbes' basic idea in developing a philosophical basis for the minimalist ethic they have called 'libertarianism'. This, despite its name, has little in common with older concepts of 'liberalism'.[17–19] Englehardt has summarised some of the assumptions of 'libertarianism' in this way:

> We . . . presuppose that not all resources and services are fully and pre-emptively state owned, that decisions to tax or transfer resources should be made openly and after public discussion, that the burden of proof is on the state to show that it is morally justified in interfering with those who wish to associate and collaborate together, that freedom of choice is valued more highly than equality of outcome, and that our commitments to beneficence are limited, as reflected by the absence of a constitutional right to receive welfare services. These we take to be the broad moral assumptions of American health care policy.

In such a philosophy freedom is an absolute, a condition and not a value of morality. It can, therefore, not be traded in the 'market place of values'. What results is a minimalist ethic, the only two requirements of which are respect for freedom and the keeping of contracts which have been freely entered into. Beneficence is supererogatory: it may be 'nice' to be beneficent but it is an aesthetic niceness and has no moral force. In a pluralist world people are said to be 'moral strangers' who know about each other merely that they want to be free to pursue their own lives in their own way.[20]

If one were to adopt such a world view entirely one could not tax the wealthy to benefit the poor, could not pass legislation designed to ensure decent food, or safe drugs, and could not license or control professionals. On such a view, being poor or ill may be undesirable and unfortunate, but it is not unjust and is no-one else's moral concern.[21] If one adheres to such a world view, the market becomes a proper instrument for trading all goods and services including health care and education. Indeed, it is the market which quite properly not only distributes commodities, but which actually underpins morality.[20]

Competition, Technology, the Market and Health Care

The market is based on several presuppositions. When these are met, the market can indeed function so as to allow consumers not only wide choice but also the ability to maximise their own values and to get what is for them the best product at the most reasonable price. Indeed, as consumers vote with their wallets and buy or refrain from buying goods, producers are stimulated to produce ever better and less expensive goods so as to attract more business to themselves. Not only are consumers thus able to buy what they consider to be the best and most reasonably priced pears, automobiles, vacations or suits of clothing but also they can choose whether to forgo one so as to buy another commodity: they can, for example, not go on vacation and instead buy a new car. To function, a market needs a large base of consumers who (1) have sufficient funds to enter the market; (2) are sure of what they want and need and are able to judge quality and price according to a standard; and (3) can take enough time to deliberate, compare and 'shop around'. When such minimal conditions are met, markets can function well and to the benefit of all.

In the US today (and in the foreseeable future) the market will control the distribution as well as the cost of health care. While under most plans proposed all citizens would receive basic medical care, they would do so under a tiered system in which insurance companies' competition (managed or otherwise) and the market will continue to be responsible for controlling costs.

As I mentioned earlier, one of the main causes of spiralling health care costs is the proliferation and misuse of technology. Modern technology, a blessing when used judiciously, has become increasingly and alarmingly expensive. Although outcome statistics for the various disease states in which major technology is used are not significantly different in countries of the industrialised Western world, the frequency and the way in which technology is used differ markedly.

The Dynamics of Technology

It is my contention that technology and its use develops its own dynamics within the free market. Magnetic resonance imagers (MRIs) have made an unquestionable contribution to today's state of the art: they are also very expensive. Competition among health care systems and providers in the US has caused a proliferation of these machines far beyond their clinical usefulness. The medium to small city in which I live, for example, has more MRIs than all of Norway, and the city of Chicago has more than all of Australia. Every medium-sized hospital, and many small hospitals, have at least one such machine, and many have several. In various cities throughout the country, such machines have been used in television and newspaper advertisements touting the superiority of one hospital over another. In many areas, furthermore, there are private entrepreneurs with free-standing units; these are often owned wholly or in part by physicians who then, of course, refer patients to such units.

Not only have the machines themselves increased in numbers: but as their numbers increase, so does their use. Their owners need to amortise their purchase and are thus interested in seeing that its use is maximal instead of optimal. The concern is, in small or large part, more the money than the information which can be derived. As lay persons hear and see about the 'wonders of science' which these machines represent, they in turn exert pressure on their physician to order such tests. Patients consulting their physician because of headaches or back-pain rarely escape without having an MRI taken. In part this is because physicians directly or indirectly profit by ordering an MRI, in part because patients demand the test, and in part because physicians fear legal suits and hope that by ordering such tests they can protect themselves. And as more such tests are ordered and more machines are purchased, the pressure to use them also increases. A story, unfortunately not rare, may illustrate the point. One of the very finest internists at our university saw a patient with what on brief history evidently were cluster headaches: a form of headache which can be easily diagnosed and treated without the use of an MRI, one indeed, in which an MRI contributes nothing. The patient had previously had an MRI ordered twice by physicians (who, however, failed to take a history!). To give another example: positronemission tomography (PET scanning) has proven to be an important research tool. Thus far its clinical use is, at best, a limited one. Nevertheless, its use in clinical medicine has often pre-empted its use in research. Far from lowering overall costs, the market has served to increase costs, demand and inappropriate usage.

What has been said about hardware can likewise be claimed for procedures. Coronary bypass surgery, for example, is far more frequently done (and the overall results in treating ischaemic heart disease are not better) in the US than it is in other parts of the Western world. Likewise, back surgery as well as some other procedures are acknowledged to be vastly over-used. The simplistic answer is that the reason for this is basically greed. While greed plays an indubitable role, such procedures (just as in the use of technology) have their own dynamics. Use is driven by the standard of care and the standard of care is, to a significant extent, driven by the market.

When competition and the market are used to 'regulate' health care, technology, instead of being used to benefit patients, is apt to be used primarily to maximise individual profit: it becomes a weapon in what is often painted as 'warfare' among health care providers and institutions. Indeed, the language of war is the language often used when competition among health care providers is discussed. This state of affairs is, I believe, based on an undue emphasis upon the demands of individual freedom to the detriment of the community. In a libertarian frame of reference, refraining from harming each other directly is the only limit society can enforce; individual choice and contract become the way all else is regulated. A market view of the world emerges in which the market, instead of being judiciously used in areas in which it has been shown to work, is used universally to distribute goods and services whether it works or not.

Health care and education, however, lend themselves but poorly to a market model. As I have said, markets, to function well, must operate under certain conditions. When it comes to health care and education, such conditions are not met. Health care and education are, as Daniels argues, 'special' in that both are needed so that people can avail themselves of the 'fair opportunity range' society offers: health care to maintain 'normal species function' and education to enable people to attain their particular goals.[22,23] People must have their biological needs met: they cannot be allowed to starve, go homeless or freeze to death. These 'first order necessities' are things that a just society, able to supply them, must guarantee its members.[24] Beyond this, it can be argued that health care and education are so critically important (they are what I have called 'second order necessities') that a society must also seek to make them freely available to all.[24] Once the means of purchase have been assured, obtaining food and shelter can be left to market forces: individuals know broadly what they want and how they are willing to spend their money. Health care (and in many respects education) are quite different: consumers are largely ignorant of what they need, are unable to judge quality and price according to a reliable standard, often are ill (sometimes desperately), coerced by fear and unable to deliberate or 'shop around'; and they can't afford to make a mistake: after all, their health or life are at stake. Choosing between health care and other social goods (say vacations), furthermore, is only an option for the healthy and fairly wealthy. When one's health or life are at stake, meaningful choice no longer exists. Furthermore, health care is so expensive that those who are not insured or very wealthy cannot enter the market at all.

Alternative Approaches

There is an alternative vision of community and ethics besides those which, at one extreme see 'community' as constituted merely to assure maximal freedom for all (and which, therefore, have a minimal effect) and, at the other extreme, which emphasise 'community' so much that it stifles all individuality. I have in mind an alternative approach to balancing individual with communal interests, an approach which is based neither on a predominance of one with neglect of the other, nor on a dialectic balance between them, but one which sees both as modifying forces in a complex homeostatic balance.

Adam Smith, often perceived as the father of today's capitalist market system, thought far beyond the market. To Adam Smith, as later to Rousseau, sympathy was conceived as basic for human nature and as initiating moral judgement. Humans, to Smith as distinct from Hobbes, are necessarily social creatures who are affected by the misfortune of others.[25] This notion appears with great strength in Rousseau's work with its emphasis on a 'primitive sense of pity' which gives rise to *'la répugnance naturelle'* to see the suffering of others. This sense (also termed compassion by Rousseau: *'l'impulse intérieure de la compassion'*) is, I believe, rightly held to be the *'Triebfeder'* or driving force of ethics by Schopenhauer.[26-28] To Rousseau, ethics was social: a product of the social contract and of the particular way in which society had constituted itself. Still, however, Rousseau saw individuals (who were for him, unlike Hobbes, amoral beings and not beings seeking to injure each other) as ontologically prior to community.

I have claimed that the discussion of whether individuals are prior to community or communities prior to individuals is a 'chicken and egg' question: unanswerable and ultimately irrelevant.[23,29] Community and individual are, like cause and effect, a word pair: one can define one only in terms of the other. Individuals who at birth, and for a few months thereafter, cannot dissociate their being from the world around them, are of necessity dependent upon nurture. Without nurture individual persons can never begin to realise their individual being. Even after they realise their individuality, continued nurture is needed if autonomy is to be attained. Throughout our lives we are, especially in a complex society, critically dependent upon the help and beneficence of others. Autonomy, far from having priority, is thus attainable only in the embrace of beneficence: in many ways, experiencing beneficence is the necessary condition for being autonomous.[23,29]

The relationship between autonomy and beneficence has often been painted as one of conflict; at best, as a dialectic tension in which each seeks to satisfy its own ends. Even if a momentary synthesis emerges from such a dialectic, it represents at best an armed truce.[29] One need not take such a view. The balance between these two forces can be seen as striving for a common goal of survival, growth and stability: a true homeostatic balance as it occurs in nature.[23] Homeostasis (whether in a cell, an organism, a species or a society) strives for sufficient balance not only to permit survival, but also to enable growth and development. The 'set-points' of such homeostasis are not rigid but adapt to external conditions. The interacting forces interact not merely to advance their own ends but, ultimately, to assure the survival essential to their own existence.[23] Far from trying to trump each other, these forces share a common interest and must, perforce, be interested in each other's goals. Individuality requires a community in which to manifest itself and communities to evolve, flourish and grow require the development of individual talents and skills. Hungry persons cannot appreciate liberty; a full stomach becomes meaningless without it.

We are not, as the libertarians claim, 'moral strangers' whose only common frame of reference is our individual desire to lead our own lives in our own way. Even when we come from quite different cultures (even, I would claim, when we belong to different but sentient species) we are bound together by at least six necessary conditions which form a framework of moral reference. We know that we all share at least:

1. A drive for being.
2. Biological needs.
3. Social needs.
4. The desire to avoid suffering.
5. A basic sense of logic (sufficient to let us recognise certain logical pre-conditions, for example that two objects cannot occupy the same space at the same time).
6. A desire to lead our own lives in our own way.

These conditions, which I have called the 'existential *a prioris* of ethics' are not principles: they are the necessary condition of existence for all sentient beings.[23] Our primitive sense of pity, our moral sentiments, allow us to recognise and value them in others. Such common conditions do not make us moral friends, but at the very least they make us moral acquaintances.

A well-functioning society recognises the needs of the individual, the needs of society and the interdependence of each with the other. In such a society, basic necessities of the first and second order will be justly distributed to all before allowing others opulence and luxury. Such a society can well use the market to distribute commodities but it will seek to place basic needs and their satisfaction beyond the market.

Allowing medical technology to be used for personal profit, rather than for the good of those who need it, distorts the balance between individual desire and communal obligation. Libertarian societies (and so stark capitalism), by giving pre-eminence to individuals and by denying beneficent obligations, defeats any meaningful solidarity and produces societies in which many will lead impoverished lives. Starkly communitarian societies (such as Bolshevism), by denigrating individuals merely to servants of the community, likewise defeat meaningful solidarity and result in impoverished lives. Neither can long endure.

References

1. Schieber, G.J., Poullier, J.P. and Greenwald, L.M. (1992). US health expenditure performance: an international comparison and update. *Health Care Financing* **13**(4), 1–88.
2. Sundstrom, P. (1994). Intensive care: who should decide? *Health Care Analysis* **2**(1), 60–64.
3. US Department of Commerce (1991). *Statistical Abstracts of the United States, 1991*. US Government Printing Office, Washington, DC.
4. US Department of Commerce (1990). *Statistical Abstracts of the United States, 1990*. US Government Printing Office, Washington, DC.
5. US Department of Commerce (1989). *Statistical Abstracts of the United States, 1989*. US Government Printing Office, Washington, DC.
6. Bernstein, A. (1989). America's income gap: the closer you look, the worse it gets. *Business Week*, 17 April 1989, 78–79.
7. Tyler, G. (1988). On the economic side. *The New Leader*, 11 July 1988, 12–13.
8. House Ways and Means Committee (1989). Cited in *New York Times*, 16 June 1989.
9. Nasar, S. (1992). Fed report gives new data on gains by richest in '80s. *New York Times*, 21 April 1992, volume CXLI (48, 943), 1 & A6.
10. Physicians Task Force on Hunger in America (1986). *Hunger in America*, Wesleyan University Press, Middletown, CT.
11. Kotlowitz, A. (1991). *There Are No Children Here: The Story of Two Boys Growing up in the Other America*, Doubleday, New York, NY.
12. Special Committee on Aging, United States Senate (1985). *America in Transition: An Aging Society*, US Government Printing Office, Washington, DC.
13. Tawney, R.H. (1954). *Religion and the Rise of Capitalism: A Historical Study*, American Library, New York, NY.
14. Hobbes, T. (1962). *Leviathan*, Collier Books, New York, NY.
15. Smith, A. (1948). An inquiry into the nature and causes of the wealth of nations. In, *Adam Smith's Moral and Political Philosophy*, ed. by H.W. Schneidr, Hafner Publishing Co, New York, NY.
16. Minogue, K.R. (1966). Thomas Hobbes and the philosophy of absolutism. In, *Political Ideas*, ed. by D. Thompson, Penguin Books, Middlesex.
17. Nozick, R. (1974). *Anarchy, State and Utopia*, Basic Books, New York, NY.
18. Engelhardt, H.T. (1988). *The Foundations of Bioethics*, Oxford University Press,

New York, NY.

19. Engelhardt, H.T. (1991). *Bioethics and Secular Humanism*, Trinity Press International, Philadelphia, PA.

20. Engelhardt, H.T. (1988). Morality for the medical–industrial complex: a code of ethics for the mass marketing of health care. *New England Journal of Medicine* **319**(16), 1086–1089.

21. Engelhardt, H.T. (1981). Health care allocation; response to the unjust, the unfortunate and the undesirable. In, *Justice and Health Care*, ed. by E.E. Shelp, D. Reidel, Dordrecht, The Netherlands.

22. Daniels, N. (1985). *Just Health Care*, Cambridge University Press, New York, NY.

23. Loewy, E.H. (1993). *Freedom and Community: the Ethics of Interdependence*, State University of New York Press, Albany, NY.

24. Loewy, E.H. (1990). Commodities, needs and health care. A communal perspective. In, *Changing Values in Medicine and Health Care Decision Making*, ed. by U.J. Jensen and G. Mooney, John Wiley and Sons, Chichester.

25. Smith, A. (1982). *The Theory of Moral Sentiments*, ed. by A.L. Macfie and D.D. Raphael, Rose Printing Company Inc., Tallahassee, FL.

26. Rousseau, J.J. (1972). *Du Contrat Social*, ed. by R. Grimsley, Oxford University Press, Oxford.

27. Rousseau, J.J. (1965). *Discours sur l'Origine et les Fondements de l'Inegalité parmi les Hommes*, Gallimard, Paris, France.

28. Schopenhauer, A. (1986). Preisschrift über die Grundlage der Moral. In, *Arrtus Schopenhauer, Sämtliche Werke, Band III* Suhrkamp, Frankfurt a/M, Germany.

29. Loewy, E.H. (1991). *Suffering and the Beneficient Community: Beyond Libertarianism*, State University of New York Press, Albany, NY.

Chapter 12

Communitarian Illusions: Or Why the Dutch Proposal for Setting Priorities in Health Care Must Fail

Theo van Willigenburg

Center for Bioethics and Health Care, Faculty of Theology, Utrecht, The Netherlands

The amount that could be spent on health care is, in theory, unlimited. We all, as mortal beings, tend to put the highest value on good health and a long life. It is true that many of the public recognise some of the problems of health care cost, but at the same time they want more rather than less medical care and are apt to demand the best available technology. Public expectations continue to grow, while expensive medical technology rapidly proliferates.

In The Netherlands, since the beginning of the 1980s, the government has tried to moderate expenditure on health care by means of various cost-containment programmes. Notable among these is a budget system where hospitals receive a lump sum, every year, based on payment forecasts, and limited by macro-budgetary constraints. This system has proved to be successful in tempering the annual increase in health care costs, but at the same time it has led to an enormous growth of waiting lists, with lengthy waiting times for many forms of health care. For example, currently the waiting time for a bed in a home for mentally handicapped persons may be up to 8 years, and many people die on waiting lists before life-saving therapy can be made available. The threat of underservice and erosion of quality is everywhere.

At the end of the 1980s it was increasingly recognised that implicit rationing through limiting the resources available to hospitals and institutes is not enough. Planned resource allocation requires the courage to set priorities. In

Reforming Health Care: The Philosophy and Practice of International Health Reform.
Edited by D. Seedhouse. © 1995 John Wiley & Sons Ltd.

The Netherlands a basic insurance programme is being introduced which will cover a large part of normal health care, so the resource allocation issue has hardened to the question: which services should be included in the basic package and which should not? What kind of services should be supplied to everyone, and which should be positioned at the bottom of the priority list?

Criteria are necessary to set priorities, and should provide good reasons in support of any distinctions made between services. Such distinctions are of greatest importance to explain the difference between services which are recommended as part of the basic package, and those which are not. The Dutch government Committee on Choices in Health Care has tried to develop criteria for setting priorities, in particular by formulating a notion of *necessary health care*. In contrast to the Oregon experiment this notion is not derived from a survey of the preferences of the population, but is based on one particular perspective on health and the purpose of health care. The government Committee has proposed a 'community-oriented perspective' from which health is seen as the possibility for every member of society to function normally and, thus, to participate as much as possible in the community.

In this article I present a brief exploration of this community-oriented approach, and investigate the validity of the notion of necessary (or essential) care.

Necessary Health Care

According to the community-oriented approach, care is necessary 'when it enables an individual to share, maintain and if possible to improve his/her life together with other members of the community'.[1] But the central question is 'which care is necessary to sustain community involvement'?

The government Committee feels that the most necessary facilities are those which guarantee 'normal functioning' or which simply protect a person's existence as a member of the community (see ten Have, Chapter six). More interesting, however, than the question of which services should be included is the question, which services are to be excluded from the basic package because they are 'not necessary enough'? The effectiveness of the community-oriented criterion of necessity depends on its power to exclude. The government Committee mention *in vitro* fertilisation (IVF) as an example of non-essential care, because undesired childlessness in The Netherlands 'poses no danger to the community, and it cannot be said that childlessness interferes with normal functioning in our society'.[1] But this is a curious argument. First, it may be said of many diseases that they are 'no danger to the community'. According to such a definition only the fight against very serious, infectious diseases might be categorised as necessary. Second, it seems to state *in general* that childlessness does not interfere with normal functioning in society. For some childless couples the impossibility of having children is an unbearable load in their life which seriously hinders their normal social functioning. Does the Dutch government Committee really think that it is possible to determine *on a macro-level* which diseases or needs interfere with normal functioning? Is it possible to determine on a macro-level whether, for instance, a motion sickness, a skin disease or a certain allergy threatens a person's normal functioning? It is hard to see how such issues can be determined without taking into account the unique situation of the individual patient. For some patients psoriasis may be a blockade to any participation in social life. Others may have learned to live with their disease. The idea of 'normal functioning', therefore, hardly seems effective as a method to determine what is essential care.

Moreover, even if it can be argued that a particular class of handicaps or diseases interferes with normal functioning it is not at all clear that it can be determined, in general, which particular health care provisions are then necessary. For instance, if we agree that a mental handicap interferes with normal functioning in society, is it possible to determine in general what kind of care for the mentally handicapped is necessary in order to enable an individual to share his life with others? What care is more necessary: 24 hour institutional care or part-time care, day-time activities or home care?

Callahan's Trap

Why has the Dutch government Committee chosen a community-oriented approach which offers such powerless criteria for setting priorities? It appears that the Committee has walked into a trap which philosophers like Daniel Callahan have been setting during recent years. The Choices in Health Care Committee rejects the approach which connects health to personal autonomy. It also rejects the 'medical professional' approach since this offers a limited definition of health in biological terms while neglecting psychosocial functioning. According to the Committee, on these theories man is perceived too much as an individual organism and not enough as a member of the social community which determines what is 'good' functioning. Leaving 'individualistic atomism' behind, the Committee embraces a more communitarian approach inspired by Callahan's ideas.[2] According to Callahan, the great problems in health care, especially the problem of the allocation of scarce resources, will remain unmanageable if society does not try to find specific answers to broad normative questions like: 'What makes a good and fulfilled life?', 'What is the place of illness and old age in our life?' and 'How may health care contribute to the good life?' Callahan is critical of the strictly liberal approach which assumes that each individual should determine what the good life is. It is essential, according to Callahan, that a community perspective on 'the good life' is developed which transcends the individual perspective. Without this no good reasons can be produced for setting priorities in health care.

Now, it may be essential, at least in Callahan's opinion, to attempt to develop a normative vision on a macro-level, but is it really possible? The Committee's proposal is a good example of what happens if one tries. In order to develop a criterion of essential care which transcends individual preferences but which may still be acceptable to different individuals, the committee gives a very broad and vague definition of health in terms of 'normal functioning', which is hardly effective as a starting point if decisions are to be prioritised. In order to make a communitarian approach practicable the meaning of 'community', 'participation in community' and 'normal functioning' must be clearly and substantially defined.

Even a minimal consensus seems hardly attainable in our pluralistic, diverse and atomistic society. That is not to say that a communitarian approach is impossible, only that our modern societies are not—in any sense—the communities of which the communitarian philosophy speaks. If this hypothetical community is postulated then either one will preach substantial normative visions which are not acceptable to many people, or one will end up with a 'community-oriented' approach which is too vague to have the necessary steering power to exclude unnecessary health care.

Back to the Primary Process

What basis do we have, then, on which to develop criteria for setting priorities in allocating health care resources? On the macro-level there is hardly such a basis, and this means that we need to return to the level where the actual choices in health care are being made: the primary process. On the 'shop-floor' in hospitals and institutions each day thousands of allocation decisions are made. Decisions which cost a lot of money and which have a direct psychological and sociological impact. The only way to develop enough steering power to get reasonable control over these processes of day-to-day health care allocation is to try to understand the history, laws, habits and contingencies of these processes. In trying to understand what is going on between doctors and patients it is, however, of little help to describe the reality of the decision-making process at the micro-level in terms of an 'individual' or 'medical professional' approach, as the Dutch government committee does. The Committee sketches the individual approach as being identical to 'the customer is always right', and it pictures the medical professional approach as 'the clinician is always right'. This has little sense. It is a pity that the Committee did not try to transcend the simple consumerist and 'medico-biological' picture, while also eschewing an appeal to the impotent communitarian approach. This would have been possible by stressing the quality of the doctor–patient relationship. Not an individual and professional approach next to each other, but a relational aproach which does not focus on the individual demand or the objective medical supply, but which stresses the importance of the biography of the patient and the way in which health care may contribute to this biography. A relational approach would also notice the biographical involvement of the health care provider who has to translate the want of the patient in a particular form of care. According to a relational approach, health care, should be provided on the basis of a mutual determination through dialogue of what care is necessary. Not necessary from an 'individual consumer' or 'medico-biological' perspective, but a necessity determined by critical doctors and well-informed patients. A broad discussion in society about the limits of necessary care may, of course, provide for a loose framework within which particular decisions are to be taken. But this does not mean that cost-containment can reasonably be reached by setting priorities on a macro-level. For, on a macro-level no powerful criteria for prioritising are available, except side-criteria like effectiveness and efficiency. Real prioritising can only be reached by again trying to get a grip on what is really going on in the primary process.

References

1. Ministry of Welfare, Health and Cultural Affairs (1992). *Choices in Health Care*, A Report by the Government Committee on Choices in Health Care, Zoetermeer, The Netherlands.
2. Callahan, D. (1987). *Setting Limits. Medical Goals in an Ageing Society*, New York, Simon and Schuster, and (1990). *What Kind of Life? The Limits of Medical Progress*, New York, Simon and Schuster.

Chapter 13

Who Should Be Responsible for a Nation's Health?

Viola Schubert-Lehnhardt

Martin-Luther Universitat Halle Wittenberg, Germany

Introduction

The movement from the socialist system to the free market system in Eastern Europe is generating deep changes in social structures, and is causing the re-examination of several social values. Developments in the former East Germany, following German unification in October 1990, are typical of the process. One of the most rapid transformations occurred in the health care system. After the unification of Germany, indeed practically 'overnight', former East German habits and practices could no longer exist.

Most former East Germans were quite unprepared for the changes. Where previously they could rely on the paternalism of the state for their health protection, they now have to act on their own initiatives. For many commentators the collapse of socialism has been unequivocally good. However, such judgements ignore the many practical difficulties caused by the upheavals. More seriously still, they disregard the fact that an entire culture has been pushed to one side, as if it has no value. In this chapter I raise the question: who should be responsible for a nation's health? Currently it is widely assumed that responsibility should always fall on the individual. However, no system is perfect and, equally, no system can be entirely bad.

Possible Bases of Responsibility

It might be argued that there are three possible bases of responsibility for health: the individual and his/her family, the professional worker (physicians, social workers and the system which supports them) and the community (a town, a region, or a state). The ethical problems that arise during settled times

Reforming Health Care: The Philosophy and Practice of International Health Reform.
Edited by D. Seedhouse. © 1995 John Wiley & Sons Ltd.

over the importance accorded to each level have been greatly emphasised by the change from the socialist to the free market system.

I shall concentrate on two aspects of the changes in Germany, and shall describe first the way 'responsibility for health' is understood in socialism.

Then, using East Germany as an example, I shall show some practical consequences of the 'overnight' break with the old traditions and habits.

The Socialist Understanding of Responsibility for Health*

In socialism both the common interpretation of 'responsibility' and the special case of 'responsibility for health' are associated with the 'marxist' image of man,† and the way in which the relationship between the individual and wider society is understood under this philosophy. A central, governing assumption of socialism is the belief that the main interests of all members conform. From this it follows that society, or at least government, has the right to create norms and values for all citizens.

Governmental control of the health care system under socialism is a prime example of this philosophy in action. Comprehensive care, managed by government, brought with it the belief that 'responsibility for health' was first and foremost a task for the state. The existence of such large-scale, centrally organised projects as medical and dental check-ups for children and adults, and the obligation to be inoculated reinforced this view of the locus of responsibility.

As a result, in health care as well as more generally, central control tended to foster disinterest, and led ultimately to the disbanding of the *societe civile* (the active sphere for citizens independent of government). Lack of initiative and denial of responsibility became permanent aspects of socialist development.[1] Yet this was not always simply a consequence of apathy. Often willing people were actually prevented from exercising responsibility, and even existing initiatives (including for example, self-help and patients' groups) were forbidden, or at least handicapped by government.

Socialist society spurned such projects, for ideological reasons, they were seen as dangerous, and certainly not as opportunities for the citizens. The few initiatives which were able to arise did so under the protection of the churches.[2] Outside the formal health care system the same situation applied to citizens movements for 'a healthy environment', special provision and accommodation for handicapped people, and construction of playgrounds (instead of car parks), to give but a few examples. Consequently, in socialism as it was practised up to 1990, individuals lacked any motive for subjective and intersubjective activities. Such was the extent of this 'enforced apathy' that their theoretical and practical autonomy was often eliminated.[3]

---

* As in the Western countries so in the Eastern ones different view points and regulations have existed. For example, a private sector existed in socialist Hungary. However, I describe here the main tendency in the postsocialist countries, using examples from the GDR.

† I put the term 'marxist' in inverted commas because a lot of ideas which were called 'marxist' by socialist authors were just the opposite of the original ideas of Karl Marx. But I do not deal with this matter here.

In health care this state of affairs built up a 'mentality of claim', and a prevalent point of view that medical care was a 'natural right'—a situation further encouraged by a vacuum of information and relevant personal experience. It is no surprise that this outlook often created risky life-styles because people were confident that they would be rescued in case of harm.

The Consequences of the 'Overnight' Break with these Old Traditions and Habits

In former East Germany young mothers now often leave hospital without necessary inoculations and check-ups for newborn children because they simply do not know that now they have to ask for these things. In former times this was done 'automatically' by the hospital personnel. Physicians are afraid that diseases which were thought to have been eradicated (for example, poliomyelitis) could arise again. Furthermore, check-ups for children and teenagers made regularly (and free of charge) in former times are not now 'demanded' by the parents. Thus it is likely that preventable problems will be recognised too late and may be dealt with either at a greater cost, or not at all.

Adults used to be called up by postcards from health care organisations for routine check-ups, X-rays, and inoculations. Under 'the new rules' everybody has to ask for these things himself, and there is no punishment. In the old system the punishment you might get if you did not follow the order was written on the postcard: I do not know of anyone actually being punished, but this doctrinaire approach certainly had a strong influence on uptake.

Because it is often no longer possible to do check-ups during working time adults do not participate in prophylactic investigation as much as before. It is commonly said that prophylactic cures and in-time-care of small injuries are not taken because people are afraid of loosing their salary or job. Or it may be once again that people simply do not know the procedures for 'demanding' such measures, which were previously provided as a matter of course. On top of this, health care is no longer free.

Presently in Germany there is widespread discussion about health care reform. In a 'united Germany' both private and state health care systems exist. The state system has 'core services' which are state funded and planned. Health care reforms are presently under discussion, and one of the main considerations concerns which services should be included in the 'core services'. But as yet no firm conclusion has been reached.

Another central debate concerns what should be free and what should be paid for, but it should not be readily assumed that paying for health care necessarily leads to better attitudes by individual people towards their own health. In many cases now the individual has to make her own decision about the level of quality she wants (that is, she must decide how much she is prepared or able to pay, even for such essentials as new dentures). Because people are not prepared for the use of the 'new autonomy' they often do not see it as something to be valued at all, and in Germany many former East German people are not equipped to make such decisions.

The cessation of the compulsory preventative measures of fluoridation of drinking water and iodation of table salt povides a further example. Here it can be seen that better preventive thinking and acting does not necessarily follow from the values of freedom and self-determination alone. In the GDR, for example, with the use of iodised salt in private and communal kitchens the figures for thyroid disease amongst newly born children fell from 12% to 1% in the 1980s. Amongst teenagers the frequency fell by up to 50% and amongst adults by about 10%. In West Germany the right to 'free decision by the user' has not produced equivalent success. Here 6% of the newborn have a goitre—and as a whole Western Germany is in last place in the European 'league-table'.[3]

People in the GDR have had to live with a lot of shortages. Only a few of them could become rich. But at the same time unemployment and homelessness were considered unreasonable. Now they have greater freedom to succeed.

However, desired results do not follow automatically from the change from a paternalistic health care system to a system founded on the idea of individual autonomy. And in making such a change a lot is lost. For example, when socialist policy disappears then so too does better social justice, solidarity and feelings of security[4]—all of which arise out of a health care system independent of the financial circumstances of individuals.[5] It should also be remarked that this 'autonomy' often is only a fictitious notion.

Freedom and self-determination in a free market system (including the 'free market for health care') are always ruled by the laws and principles of this system. This means that freedom of choice is often only a freedom for the person who has the financial means to pay for his chosen means.

During the rapid unification of Germany the advantages and disadvantages of both systems were not equally evaluated and taken as a basis for the new system. On the contrary only one system, with its particular values and principles, was taken as the model for the other one. The colonialism may have been enthusiastic, but it was also disrespectful.

References

1. Kellner, E. and Soldan, A. (1991). Die Reduktion des Individuums—Versuch einer Auseinandersetzung mit der realsozialistischen Ethik. *Deutsche Zeitschrift für Philosophie* **39**(4), 433.
2. A description of this situation is given in: Selbsthilfegruppen—Entwicklungen in der DDR. Nakos.extra. Juli, 1990.
3. See the studies which are evaluated in: 'Staatlich verordnete Salzjodierung' in der DDR liess Strumaerkrankungen zurückgehen. Jetzt geraten alle guten Ergebnisse in Gefahr. Neues Deutschland vom 31.3.1991.
4. Luther, E. (1991). Wie konsensfähig ist eine maxistisch orientierte medizinische Ethik? In, *Grundfragen Medizinischer Ethik in der Diskussion*, ed. by V. Schubert-Lehnhardt, Halle.
5. Schubert-Lehnhardt (1993). Medicine and Justice In *Ethik zwischen Anspruch und Wirklichkeit*, June 27 1992 in Halle.

Chapter 14

A Turn for the Better? Philosophical Issues in Evaluating Health Care Reforms

Alan Cribb

Centre for Educational Studies, King's College London, UK

How can we evaluate something as large and indeterminate as health care reform? There are certainly many methodological difficulties. Reforms entail a complex of interacting changes, intended and unintended, coherent and conflicting. Many factors 'outside' health care affect health care and health. Tracing cause and effect is almost impossible. But there are also fundamental philosophical difficulties. Given that we can broadly describe the changes, how can we ascribe value to them? What sort of things make health care valuable? These are important questions which ought to be dominating public debate about health care reforms. If we do not ask them there is a danger that health care reform will be evaluated by inappropriate criteria; that policy makers will wake up to the concerns of professionals and clients, and the limitations of specific reforms, when it is too late to reverse the damage. In what follows I will argue that the recent 'internal market' reforms of the UK health service represent a serious threat to the care it offers, and that this threat may be missed by dominant models of evaluation. My argument rests on a consideration of 'evaluation' which I will set out first; including a distinction between 'extrinsic' and 'intrinsic' evaluation, and a discussion of the interactions between social contexts and social relations. Although this framework is used here to raise some concerns about specific reforms it is intended to be of wider relevance.

Reforming Health Care: The Philosophy and Practice of International Health Reform.
Edited by D. Seedhouse. © 1995 John Wiley & Sons Ltd.

Extrinsic and Intrinsic Evaluation

We can treat a health care system like a black box and look at 'the inputs' and 'the outputs', or we can focus on the contents of the box. I shall call these two approaches extrinsic and intrinsic evaluation. I should say at once that this distinction is far from clear-cut; it is difficult to determine what falls inside or outside the system, which things are outputs and which processes, but we will return to this. One reason to adopt this distinction is that something like it is presupposed in much health care analysis. The ideas of 'health outcomes', 'health gain', or 'cost-effectiveness' are very often employed as if a health care system was merely a means of converting money into some other commodity. By contrast the growth in the 'quality' literature is partly an attempt to capture something of the process and experience of care (although some authors use 'outcomes' and 'quality' almost interchangeably).

How far is it possible to separate out extrinsic from intrinsic evaluation? If we are dealing with entirely mechanical or technological processes then it seems perfectly possible. We can judge how well a particular function is performed and at what cost. Efficiency is the watchword, and it is a key element of extrinsic evaluation. Here the box contains no ethical objects or social relations and so there is no question of intrinsic ethical evaluation. In the normal case the functioning of an electricity generator can be more or less efficient, but it cannot, in itself, be more or less ethical. (Of course it may be unethical for someone to *use* a wasteful generator.) But if the generator works on animal or human power things alter. We can still ask about efficiency—a generator that produces the same wattage from two people rather than four is 'better'—but other issues arise, e.g. questions of kindness, fairness, etc. Yet we still might try to separate out extrinsic from intrinsic evaluation. Take a slave-based society: we can evaluate the contribution of the institution of slavery to the 'productivity' of society, and this is quite different from asking whether it can be reformed so as to make it less intolerable to the slaves.

Let us take some other cases. Imagine a penal system in which convicted criminals are forcibly injected with chemicals which make them law abiding but (miraculously) have no side-effects. Or a military academy in which young soldiers are taught with 'student-centred' methods how to torture. In all these cases one or other type of evaluation seems to determine the issue. If there is something plainly wrong with either the means or the ends then the whole institution is put in doubt. This does not take us very far, but perhaps it is still worth stating: any reform of a health care system which turns health workers into 'slaves' or makes them engage in ethically unacceptable practices should be put in doubt, even if it results in great gains in efficiency and passes other standards of extrinsic evaluation. This provides a crude picture of a limit to reforms, and it may also serve as a useful piece of rhetoric for those who wish to emphasise their hostility to the effects of certain health reforms.

But there are relatively few instances of consensus about 'the plainly wrong'. (Even some of the above examples may fail to fit the bill.) Using it as the 'litmus test' by which to assess health care reforms is not a promising approach. Social relations are complex and multi-faceted, and are subject to contestable characterisations which embody competing value perspectives. Any judgements that they (or their aspects or effects) are ethically unacceptable are likely to be hotly disputed.

Social Relations and their Institutional and Social Context

Consider marriage: some see it as the cornerstone of civilisation and morality, others as a form of social oppression and division. In both these cases it is difficult to disentangle extrinsic from intrinsic evaluation, but once again we can try. Advocates of marriage on the basis of its perceived social benefits are likely to hesitate before judging particular marriages to be intrinsically bad, but this is a judgement that they can make. Similarly someone who regards marriage as patriarchal and exploitative may still believe that particular marriages are, in themselves, not too bad. In an age of sociological awareness we are often uncomfortable and self-conscious about the tensions revealed in these judgements. We know, for example, that particular marriages and the institution of marriage are mutually supporting and that in endorsing one we are indirectly supporting the other. Indeed social relations are partly constituted by their institutional and social context, and vice versa. Here is another reason for the distinction between intrinsic and extrinsic evaluation to weaken or break down.

Thus to the extent that we can differentiate between 'inside' and 'outside' an institution (or a set of relations) we must also consider the interactions between the two. We might, to pick one of many possible metaphors, talk of 'contamination' of one by the other. Or we might talk about attempts to 'insulate' social relations from their social context. Similarly we can talk about contamination or insulation between the ways of thinking and talking appropriate to extrinsic and intrinsic evaluation. If health care is seen as a black box—we can (1) look at the inputs and the outputs, or (2) look at the social relations within the box. But we must also consider (3) the questions of insulation and contamination. In what follows I want to say something about each of these things but I will concentrate mainly on the last as it is often neglected.

These considerations suggest that it might be better to drop the false separation of extrinsic and intrinsic, of outputs and processes, for a unified perspective and language of evaluation. But both empirical and philosophical problems attach to this. As a matter of fact much evaluation of health care concentrates on a single limited perspective, often on outputs such as the number of people treated over a unit of time, or for a unit of resource. Although it is possible to collect more subtle and more complex data this is at the expense of less measurable and more contestable interpretations. These facts about empirical research reflect underlying philosophical issues—above all the problem of monism versus pluralism. There appear to be a number of qualitatively different goods (in general, and in relation to health care) which can only be captured by different ways of talking. Even if we concentrate on health care outputs (or 'health gain') then (1) there are many relevant goods (e.g. life, comfort, vigour, self-esteem, etc.), and (2) different methods of accounting these goods, i.e. the languages of economic efficiency and distributive justice both apply but do not seem reducible one to the other. (The push for monism partly arises from the inescapable need for overall evaluation—we have, for example, to choose policy A or B, state of affairs A or B—but the need for an overall judgement does not entail that there is a single over-arching language.)

Let us—for the sake of argument—see the health care box as containing something like the actions and social relations which constitute health care (within the health care system), i.e. relations between health professionals, and between health professionals and clients. It is possible to see intrinsic evaluation as the business of mainstream health care ethics and the philosophy of health; whereas extrinsic evaluation tends to revolve around economic and political questions about efficiency and equity. Most political and economic analysis takes place without reference to health care ethics. Similarly discussions in health care ethics frequently ignore the social context of professional–client relationships. This is despite the fact that the 'social construction' of health care is the focus of much sociological analysis.

The process of reform highlights the artificiality of these separations between 'macro' and 'micro' perspectives. If public policy is static, or is only shifting gently, then it can come to be viewed as the almost invisible backcloth against which the processes of health care can be studied. Once public policy is subject to substantial reform its interpenetration with care becomes striking. (Some reforms partly consist of increasing the interpenetration of policy and care.) Perhaps the most frequently cited example of this is the debate about rationing. Here is an issue which obviously connects macro and micro decision-making. In many ways it exemplifies the concerns I want to explore. I will briefly illustrate these concerns with reference to the familiar example of rationing. But it is not (or not primarily) the substantive issues of rationing that are of interest to me here but all of the factors which shape 'the culture of care'.

It is often observed that rationing goes on, by necessity, in all health care systems; and that the high profile of this topic has come to have in recent health policy largely amounts to making explicit previously 'hidden contests and judgements'. Indeed many people argue that increased openness or transparency is in itself an important step forward. Although I do not want to deny the advantages of transparency it is possible to attach a cost, and perhaps a very high cost, to its wholesale pursuit. In short, if every health care relationship is seen by everyone, including those involved, as an exercise in rationing then the nature of the relationship, and the nature of care, may be changed profoundly for the worse.

Rationing aims at the efficient use of resources. Health economists are right to stress that efficiency is neither amoral nor non-moral but is an important element of ethical evaluation. It is wrong to waste resources on ineffective interventions, and at least up to a point it makes sense to distribute resources so as 'to do most good'. (This is not the place to review these arguments.) However this utilitarian way of thinking can, notoriously, come into conflict with the orientation of much traditional health care ethics. (Later I will say more about the idea of 'traditional' health values.)

If we want to evaluate a push for efficiency we could look at it extrinsically and ask whether it has actually worked (resulted in greater efficiency, somehow measured) and what other 'outputs' it has had—what impact has it had on the distribution of treatment or equity? Alternatively we could look at individual health care relationships and see how they have been affected. If these latter are defined very narrowly then there may be little direct effect, i.e. *when* people are treated they may be treated in much the same way as before. However the impact on relationships may be quite direct: the same intervention may be allocated half the time, or a practitioner may be replaced with a less-experienced (and cheaper) colleague or by a computer or other tool. Finally, we could look at the indirect effects of the push for efficiency on health care relationships. How has the 'rationing' culture altered the nature of these relationships? These effects can take two forms.

1. The 'rationing' culture and the 'traditional culture' might conflict, with the former exerting pressure on the latter, thereby constraining choice and action.
2. The 'rationing culture' might colonise, and to some degree replace or transform, aspects of the traditional culture thereby altering the orientation of health workers and the nature of their relationships with each other and with clients.

The remainder of the chapter is a broader exploration of these issues, and the relationship between policy, culture and care with reference to the UK health care reforms. This is a philosophical rather than an empirical 'case study' with the aim of reviewing the dimensions of the debate rather than focusing on the details.

Evaluating UK Health Market Reforms

Efficiency is arguably the central policy objective of the recent UK health care reforms, but it is only one of a cluster of ideas which inform the reforms and which make up their ideology and rhetoric. The mechanism for resource allocation in the new NHS is an internal market in which 'providers' (mainly hospitals) compete for the (publicly funded) resources of the district health authority and GP 'purchasers' according to the NHS and Community Care Act, 1990. The market is intended to encourage efficiency through provider competition and purchaser choice, and market regulation is in place to protect and monitor rules and standards of contracting. These reforms not only amount to a radical restructuring of health service institutions, systems of funding and systems of accountability, but also they rest upon a deliberate and systematic attempt at cultural reform: the attempted introduction of an 'enterprise culture' into the public health service. Within many of the new provider organisations (e.g. hospital trusts) these attempts at cultural reform have been vigorously pursued with a re-education of all grades of staff in the language and demands of the market-place.

Hence cultural reform encompasses a number of interlocking elements: a focus on outcomes and performance indicators (characteristic of utilitarian ways of thinking), emphasis upon 'value for money' as a spur to competitive efficiency, a re-orientation of lines of accountability away from national and local democracy and towards local managers and independent boards, and a concern with legitimating services in the market-place through presentation and public relations, and through increasing the influence of 'choice' as expressed by purchasers. A competitive system demands the fostering of a competitive mentality, and clear systems of institutional incentives for treating patients efficiently.

Four historical factors make the 'internal market' reforms difficult to evaluate:

1. Despite pressure from health professionals, there were no trial schemes before the changes came into force in April 1991.
2. The government chose not to introduce any official research or monitoring of the internal market.
3. The introduction of the internal market coincided with a number of other important changes including increases in overall resourcing, new GP contracts, health promotion initiatives, and a *Patients Charter*.[1]
4. Although the reforms have been in place for a few years their introduction has been phased and closely regulated with a 'steady state' in the first year and 'managed change' thereafter. Even if change is accelerated it will be many years before the full consequences of the internal market become visible.

Yet the absence of an officially co-ordinated evaluation exercise has not prevented countless assessments of the reforms. It is impossible to talk to anyone in the health service without hearing a personal and professional evaluation of the changes they are experiencing! Amongst other things these stories remind us that it is foolish to expect the experience of change to be all good or all bad. The internal market impacts on different individuals and groups in very different ways. Power and status relations have shifted, new hierarchies have arisen. New forms of constraint and new forms of opportunity have been created. This is not the place to try and summarise or systematise this sort of evidence. But it is worth briefly reviewing the conclusions of some of the policy analysts who have collated evidence in order to provide an overall assessment of the impact of reforms. These suggest that the reforms may have performed poorly or badly even as judged by their primary objective.

Maynard's economic analysis of the introduction of competition into the NHS asks whether enhanced treatment practices will offset the costs of maintaining the new structures, and concludes that 'collaborative transactions' may be more efficient than competition. 'Indeed there remains little evidence to sustain the claims of political rhetoric that competition "works"'.[2] Not surprisingly there is a growing body of evidence that the reforms are faring even more badly so far as equity is concerned. Whitehead rehearses this evidence and argues that 'recent policies seem to be taking the NHS away from the goal of an equitable system'.[3] In particular she draws attention to the discriminatory effects of incentives introduced by the internal market reforms to select and treat patients on financial grounds rather than on the basis of need.

The most wide-ranging evaluative consideration of the reforms has been conducted by the King's Fund Institute.[4] In summary this report argues that there is, as yet, little evidence of any dramatic change, but agrees that there are 'equity worries', for example, about the growth of a two-tier service. On the other hand it sees some scope for being positive about the reforms: some studies have noted some improvements in communication—although there is considerable doubt about how far this should be attributed to the internal market reforms rather than to other changes. This cautious appraisal of the reforms should be contrasted with the judgement of the British Medical Association as expressed by its Chairman, Sandy Macara, 'Rather than improving efficiency, the reforms imposed on the NHS have increased bureaucracy, reduced patient choice, limited the range of core services, and led to inequity of treatment'.[5]

This sort of antipathy to the reforms is common amongst health professionals; those who are 'on the inside' often make severe judgements about the consequences of the reforms; why is this? It is too simple to say that they reflect vested interests which have been challenged by the changes, although there is no doubt some truth in this. A better explanation is found in some of the other concerns expressed by Macara[6] and others, about changes in the climate or culture of care:

> Co-operation has been supplanted by commercial competition. There is an uncontrolled, ill-managed internal market pitting purchaser against provider, fund-holding GP against non-fund-holding GP, GP against consultant, junior against senior, hospital against hospital and all to serve a perverse philosophy of winners and losers. Business plans override clinical priority. Money does not follow the patient: the patient has no choice but to follow the money.

Thus however uncertain we ought to be about the 'outputs' of the reforms, many health professionals judge that they are already in a position to assess their impact on the culture and social relationships which constitute health care. In essence the changes are seen to be socially divisive and corrosive, and to replace health care values with business values. Advocates of the internal market reforms might plausibly regard these perceptions as intra-professional worries springing from the pains of cultural adaptation; perceptions which will shift with continued reform and professional re-education. But these perceptions, and the feelings behind them, deserve to be taken a good deal more seriously.

Caring

Perhaps the most fundamental transformation that may result from the reforms is a transformation in the nature of care itself. The idea of commodification captures the business of 'putting a price' on patients which arises from systems of financial incentives. There are important parallels here with critiques of medicalisation. The sick person is not only transmuted into 'disease x' but also becomes 'invoice y'. Hence 'commodification' implies a shift in the nature of professional–client relationships, and in particular a reification of the client into an object: a liability or an asset. This kind of language may appear largely rhetorical; an emotive over-statement, and an over-reaction to cultural change. I am conscious of the risks, and the dangers, of over-statement but nonetheless want to argue that this project of cultural reform in the UK health service constitutes a serious threat to the nature of the care it offers.

Undoubtedly part of the widespread hostility to the UK health reforms is emotional. Many British people have a deep-seated sense of attachment to and loyalty towards, the NHS and what it has symbolised. The fact that a reaction is emotional, taken by itself, is neither a strength nor a weakness. Certainly part of the reaction might be called 'aesthetic'. There is a distaste, particularly amongst many public sector professionals, for a mixing of business and welfare values. Some of this should perhaps be discounted. A doctor who argues (as a few still seem to) that one should not even entertain economic considerations in health care is simply unrealistic. Also there may be a certain amount of snobbishness in not wanting to dirty one's hands with mere 'trade'. But behind all this there are fundamental, albeit difficult, ethical questions about the compatibility of an 'enterprise culture' with a 'caring culture'.

Much of the debate about the reform of the public sector is conducted against unexamined assumptions about motivation. It is tempting for some to suppose that health care professionals are motivated purely from concern for the welfare of others; that practical caring rests upon a generous caring disposition. On the other hand many analysts and critics have pointed to the personal ambitions of health professionals, their attachment to power and status and other extrinsic rewards. The introduction of financial and commerical factors into the health care culture in the UK does not represent the first taint of worldliness to the unworldly. Indeed there is plenty of reason to succumb to the opposite temptation: to suppose that health professionals are solely motivated by personal gain of one form or another, even (or perhaps especially) by extrinsic rewards. This simple-minded division between the selfless and the selfish (along with a common presumption that the former reduces to the latter) seems to have caught on in popular psychology, but insofar as this axis is assumed as the background to the evaluation of privatisation or marketisation it obscures as much as it clarifies. Many things we do are not, in the ordinary sense, either selfless or selfish.

Let us consider the case of friendship which is in some ways analogous to health care. I can only be your friend if our relationship is not solely instrumental. You might say that anyone who does not know this does not understand what friendship is. So if we are asked about the value of a particular friendship our answer would not be exhausted by all the favours or forms of emotional and practical support that the individuals concerned derive from one another. One way of putting this is to say that the friendship is an end in itself, or is an intrinsic good as well as an extrinsic good. This way of talking appears to transcend the altruism—egoism axis, but it also sounds mysterious or even mystical. It seems to rest upon the idea that there is value in the world which does not consist in (but may coincide with) valuable experiences for individuals. Although I think this idea is defensible, it is not necessary to settle that here. All that is necessary to establish is that there are commitments, projects and activities which have 'shared ends',[7] of which friendship is paradigmatic. That is, there are activities which are not analysable wholly in individualistic terms. Many of the things we do involve participation in shared 'practices'—for example, football or history—which are not reducible to individual outputs.[8] For many people this is a central feature of things that they consider to be most worthwhile. But to derive satisfaction from activities with shared ends is neither to be selfish nor selfless, nor is it particularly helpful to say that it is both of these things; rather the distinction breaks down in these cases.

MacIntyre makes a helpful distinction between what he calls 'internal' and 'external goods'. The latter, such as status and money, are contingently attached to practices. 'There are always alternative ways of achieving such goods, and their achievement is never to be had *only* by engaging in some particular kind of practice.' Internal goods are specific to, and inherent in, practices. We can only participate in these goods by participating in the practices of which they are part.

> It is characteristic of what I have called external goods that when achieved they are always some individual's property and possession . . . but it is characteristic of them (internal goods) that their achievement is good for the whole community who participate in the practice.[8]

There are important analogies between friendship and health care, and this is not to idealise health care relationships. Certainly there are substantial differences between the two. Health care is essentially a set of instumental and partial relationships; and the relationships which make it up are constituted and circumscribed by certain (albeit relatively open-ended) goals and tasks. Nonetheless health care is not altogether different from friendship, and on occasions it has the potential to embody qualities akin to those of friendship. First, nursing and medicine, and the other traditions which form health care are full of collective practices with shared ends. Researching, planning, organising, and delivering care are typically regarded as inherently worthwhile. Partly this is because these activities involve the collaborative development and cultivation of valued knowledge, skills and dispositions. Partly it is because these activities aim, directly or indirectly, at the well-being of actual or potential clients. Second, at least on occasions, the health care relationship itself is intrinsically worthwhile (or has value which is not necessarily translated into 'health gain' or other individual outcomes)—the ideal of professional caring or befriending has quite properly been discussed as a form of 'moderated love'.[9] Hence the value of health care is not captured by its 'outputs', where these are understood as the health benefits to specific clients or as the extrinsic rewards of specific professionals.

Loosely speaking health care provides 'health' and 'care'. To employ the false distinction once more—the former is the output and the latter the process (although it too can be *called* an output). Both faces of health care matter, and need to be considered in the evaluation of reforms. In some cases it is right to give most emphasis to the former, but very often it is the latter which is closer to the heart of the matter. For example, if we are talking about the management of chronic illness, or support for disability, or community care for the elderly, etc. then recognition and respect for the individual is the central concern. Indeed sometimes health care simply consists of one individual paying proper attention to another. To care does not mean to feel caring all the time; *feelings* of caring are susceptible to mood changes, tiredness and so on, and are not always possible or appropriate. But caring does mean to value other individuals, and our relationships with them, as ends in themselves. Health care reforms must be judged according to their tendency to facilitate, or undermine, a caring culture. Intrinsic evaluation, including 'cultural evaluation', is at least as important as extrinsic evaluation.

Contamination or Insulation?—Some Conclusions

Relationships between friends are put under threat whenever the instrumental value of one friend to another overshadows the intrinsic value of the friendship; the thought of 'being used' is incompatible with friendship. For this reason combining business relationships with friendships is notoriously problematic, and requires continual balancing acts. Is the same true of health care relationships? Will the introduction of market values, competition, and incentives into the UK health service undermine the traditional values of the service, and the nature of care?

Up to now I have written about 'traditional values' of health care as if they represent a coherent set. Of course they do not; health care ethics and philosophy of health is largely about mapping the complexities, tensions and contradictions inherent in health care values. The pre-reform NHS was shaped by competing commitments, partial commitments, and pragmatism. Egalitarian and utilitarian threads have always been tangled up with each other, and with political and professional ideologies. However, along with this complexity, the NHS can also be seen as host to a fragile 'moral tradition' (or traditions) of valuable 'practices' which embody the ideals, dispositions, and skills of caring. Part of this tradition is the continuing debate and conversation about values. In many ways internal market values represent just one more voice in this debate rather than a clear-cut challenge to it.

As we have seen, conflict between traditional values and business values is not so simple as a conflict between selflessness and selfishness. Health professionals have commitments to institutions as well as to clients. Loyalty to institutions may derive in part from self-interest, but not entirely. In a competitive market professionals' duties are structured by the need to keep their institution or unit thriving or in existence. Inevitably the financial incentives and disincentives which motivate the market become part of the culture and the mentality of professionals. The risk is that the market mentality privileges certain values over others in a way that is harmful to health care.

If health care relationships are not informed by some degree of 'economic realism' practitioners will be either wasteful or unfair. The focus on cost-effectiveness has many benefits. So when ought we to decide that 'contamination' by finance is a bad thing? As well as the factors (social divisiveness and inequity) mentioned above, there are two reasons to fear the impact of the UK internal market reforms on the tradition of care. First, these reforms appear to represent a 'thinning down' of values. Nursing, medicine and the other caring traditions provide a rich system of practical knowledge, judgements, sensitivities, checks and balances; whereas the internal market reforms place considerable emphasis on limited criteria of success and failure—such as hospital 'league tables'. Narrow forms of instrumentalism are being fostered. Second, the increased emphasis upon business decision-making has, in many instances, been accompanied by a diminution of professional autonomy. Professional autonomy is not an absolute good and has to be balanced against other concerns; but there is plenty of anecdotal evidence to suggest that many professionals feel that they are losing 'authorship' of their actions. Thus even where professionals are 'going through the same motions' they may not be *doing* the same things. The danger is that in the long term not only their morale, but also the subtlety and quality of their care will deteriorate.

Of course this does not provide a blanket excuse for bad practice. Cultures do not completely determine individual actions. The 'internal market' culture is mediated by a number of local, institutional and personal factors. There is no doubt that the traditional values of health care will be defended by professional integrity, and by professional commitment to the practices of care. But it should also be noted that there are limits to how far professionals can resist the colonisation of their institutional cultures; and that certain institutional and cultural climates are inhospitable to professional integrity.

None of the comments I have made here presuppose that a private system of health care is necessarily incapable of providing good quality care. The key question is not whether the values intrinsic to care be maintained alongside professional and institutional rewards. There is no health system, public or private, which does not depend upon these things co-existing. The key question is how can they best be maintained alongside each other. This involves a consideration of moral psychology and sociology. Can it be left to the virtues of clear-headed individuals to insulate the intrinsic from the instrumental values? More realistically, we should ask whether we can create structures and cultures which act as insulators, and which help individual professionals to strike a balance between private and public interests, and between health gain and care.

Acknowledgement

I am very grateful to my friend Sharon Gewirtz for helping me sort out my thoughts about these issues.

References

1. DOH, (1991). *The Patient's Charter*, Department of Health, HMSO, London.
2. Maynard, A. (1993). Competition in the UK National Health Service: Mission impossible? *Health Policy* 23, 193–204.
3. Whitehead, M. (1994). Who cares about equity in the NHS? *British Medical Journal* 308, 1284–1287.
4. Robinson, R. and Le Grand, J. (1994). *Evaluating the NHS Reforms*, King's Fund Institute, Newbury.

5. Macara, A.W. (1994). Reforming the NHS reforms. *British Medical Journal* **308**, 848–849.
6. Macara, A.W. (1994). Address to the BMA. *The Guardian* July 5th.
7. White, J. (1990). *Education and the Good Life*, Kogan Page, London.
8. MacIntyre, A. (1991). *After Virtue*, Duckworth, London.
9. Campbell, A. (1984). *Moderated Love*, SPCK, London.

Part Three:
The Need for Theory—A Case Study in the Philosophy of Health Promotion

Chapter 15

On the Nature and Ethics of Health Promotion. An Attempt at a Systematic Analysis

Lennart Nordenfelt

Department of Health and Society, University of Linköping, Sweden

Introduction

In this chapter I do two things. First, I suggest a taxonomy and a system for classifying various types of health promotion. In particular, I place the categories of health promotion in an action–theoretical context, taking advantage of some of the results obtained in the field of modern philosophical action theory. Second, I use this classification in discussing some major issues within the ethics of health promotion.

By health promotion I mean something very general. I incorporate all measures performed by a particular individual A with the intention of maintaining or improving the health of some other individual B, where A and B can, but need not, be identical persons. An important exception from this general characteristic is, however, made: I am not concerned with curative medical health care.

To promote health, as I see it, means intentionally trying to maintain or improve at least one person's state of health. Such measures can be of several types. One sort of classification that can be made has to do with what and how many agents are involved in the health-promotive action. First, I distinguish between *individual actions, institutional actions* and *collective actions*. An individual health-promotive action is one with only one agent. An example of this is the mother who sees to it that her son puts on a raincoat on a rainy autumn morning; another example is the teacher who advises his pupils not to smoke. By an institutional action I mean, for instance, a piece of legislation that is

Reforming Health Care: The Philosophy and Practice of International Health Reform.
Edited by D. Seedhouse. © 1995 John Wiley & Sons Ltd.

performed by an institution in its name and which has a health-promotive purpose. The institution can be of any kind; it may, for example, be a parliament, a court, a health education board or an athletics club. The main characteristic of an institutional action is that no particular person is responsible for the action (an exception being, perhaps, the case where an institution consists only of one individual). By a collective action I mean such action as presupposes at least two co-operative agents and where at least one of the participants has a health-promotive purpose with his or her action. A football match in which at least one of the players has a health-promotive purpose is an example of a collective health-promotive action.

Health-promotive actions can be more or less *direct*. By direct I mean an action which involves some direct manipulation of the object's body. It is important to realise that such actions can be undertaken outside purely medical care. I have in mind such things as vaccination and preventive surgical operations. By direct manipulation I also mean the patient's own activities with body and mind, including abstention from certain activities. The action of building a sports centre, however, can only contribute *indirectly* to health-promotive effects. The sports centre plays the role of providing the opportunity for other actions of a sports character, which in their turn can affect the health of the people involved. The original action of building the centre fulfils the condition of being a health-promotive action in my sense if it is performed with the intention of improving the health of the population. (Observe, however, that there is no requirement that the action shall be effective with respect to health for it to be called a health-promotive action.)

A particularly important type of indirect action comprises those activities which entail *interaction*, i.e. where a main agent *A* intends to influence another agent *B* to act in a certain direction in order for the latter to maintain or improve his or her level of health. This is the class of actions that generates the most interesting ethical dilemmas.

A further essential classification of health-promotive actions has to do with the varying nature of the goal of health. I have already preliminarily characterised health promotion as the action of either maintaining a state of health or improving it. This indicates that I do not regard the goal of health as an absolute state but as a gradable dimension along which every person's state of health can be placed. Within the framework of certain conceptual structures, for instance my own, this dimension has two absolute endpoints, on the one hand *maximal* or *optimal* health, and on the other hand non-existent health, which is represented by total and irreversible loss of consciousness or by death.

In order to make these specifications clearer we have to supplement this characterisation with an analysis of the notion of health. I must here bypass this analysis. I refer the reader to my publications *On the Nature of Health*[1] and *Towards a Theory of Health Promotion*.[2] Here I state only the definition which I propose, which is a holistic action-oriented notion, and not a biostatistical, purely medical one.

1. *A* is in a state of complete health, if and only if *A* has the ability, given standard circumstances, to realise all his vital goals.

2. A has some degree of illness (or non-health) if and only if A, given standard circumstances, cannot realise all his vital goals or can only partly realise them.

(For a further specification of the concepts of vital goal and standard circumstance, see the publications referred to above.)

There are two important conclusions to be drawn from accepting such a notion of health in a health-promotive context. Let me make only the most essential observations.

If a person's health consists of his or her ability to realise vital goals under standard circumstances, then health promotion must be something more than just disease prevention. The latter is still, of course, an important part of health promotion. In many instances disease prevention is a precondition of health promotion. But it is not in itself the ultimate goal.

It is also important to note that the prevention of illness (or non-health) has a wider connotation than disease prevention. Non-health (in the sense of non-ability to realise vital goals) can exist for reasons other than disease, injury or defect. It can, for instance, be the consequence of existential problems.

In both these respects the presented theory goes in the same direction as that advocated by the World Health Organisation (WHO). However, my definition is not quite as inclusive as that of the WHO.

The Various Forms of Health Promotion

I shall now make a closer analysis of some of the forms of health promotion from the point of view of their more concrete contents. I then use this analysis in my subsequent discussion of ethical problems.

I have already stated that by direct health promotion I mean a direct manipulation of the bodies of one or more persons. Manipulative somatic health care is therefore an example of such direct action. But non-curative health enhancement can also be direct. Vaccination, and the elimination of liver spots on the skin for preventive reasons are good examples of this.

However, most forms of health promotion—those which are generally discussed in the literature and which have the greatest ethical interest—have an indirect character. Their influence on a particular person is then mediated by some further causal link, either some action or some series of natural events.

Let me distinguish here between two main types of indirect health promotion.

1. Health promotion through *change of the environment*. Here the logic of action is the following. A influences the health of B by changing some part of B's physical or cultural environment. (The influence here can be even more indirect. A can try to influence someone else, for instance an authority, to decide to make a change in B's environment. This case then also involves the type of health promotion which is to be discussed below.)
2. Health promotion through *interaction*. By interactive health promotion I mean here the case where an agent A influences another agent B to perform a directly health-promotive action.

My analysis of the major cases of interaction is performed by using a model of action explaination. (This model was first presented in von Wright.[3] It was expanded and discussed in detail in Nordenfelt;[4] and also later.[2])

Behind a certain human action H, we normally have the following components:

1. A intends to realise a certain state P.
2. A judges that he is in situation S.
3. A judges that it is necessary for him to perform H in order to reach P.
4. A has the ability and opportunity to perform H.

According to the theory for this model (for which the term *practical syllogism* was coined by von Wright) these four components are sufficient to explain why the person A at a particular time performed H. (The complete model also contains some further specifications; see Nordenfelt.[4])

In a similar way one can say that if these four conditions are fulfilled, then the agent A will perform the action in the future; the four components are together *sufficient determinants* of a future action H.

This latter observation makes the model fruitful for the analysis and classification of interaction in general, and interactive health promotion in particular. One can influence the course of action of a particular person by manipulating one or more of the components of the practical syllogism, and one can manipulate various combinations of them.

In an extreme case one can imagine that an influencing agent creates or changes all four components in the model. In more realistic cases the agent deals with only one particular component. Let me illustrate with a simple example of health education.

Let us imagine that a health education board carries out research into the existence of moulds in a block of houses. It appears that the situation is serious. Most of the investigated houses are affected. The risk of contracting asthma allergy is very high, in particular for the children in the affected population. As a result the board informs the inhabitants in the block about the situation. The circumstances are described as highly dangerous to their health.

Let us now assume that most of the inhabitants already possess a determinant of action corresponding to the following:

A has the standing intention of maintaining his own good state of health.

Through the information from the board a possible component 2 is created or changed in A. A has come to know about the dangerous environment. As a result A can perhaps on his own form a component 3, i.e. decide what he must do in order to avoid the threat. Alternatively, he can be helped in this respect by the board again. They can give him advice about possible measures he might take. As a result we can have the following syllogism represented among most of the inhabitants in the block.

1. A has the intention of maintaining his health.
2. A judges that the mould situation in his house is dangerous to his health.
3. A judges that he must carry out a complete sanitation of the house (he may

for instance have to fumigate it) in order to maintain his and his family's health.

4. *A* has the financial resources and has every opportunity to realise this sanitation.

As a result of all this *A* performs the required action.

This is an analysis of a health-promotive action of the information kind. Now similar presentations can be performed for other kinds of interaction, such as recommendation, advice, threat and persuasion.

Ethical Aspects of the Various Forms of Health Promotion

The General Utility Argument for Health Promotion

In popular discussion medical ethics has often been identified as a subject which deals with ethical *problems* or ethical *dilemmas*. It is understandable why this is so. In practical affairs one has a need for an ethicist when one perceives problems, when one's own ethical intuitions do not suffice for making clear-cut decisions.

This fact should not preclude that there is a general ethical framework within which all our actions are or could be placed. All activities that we consider to be good or right must have an ethical motivation. There is always some basic ethical consideration that makes them good or right.

Health care and health promotion are no exceptions. They are considered by all to be extremely valuable enterprises. When we are asked why we set a high value on them we normally refer to some kind of utility argument. We say, for instance, that health is a value because it is a precondition for the efficient production of utilities, *or* health is a value because it is a precondition for a high degree of happiness which in itself is (one of) the ultimate human value(s).

This basic extremely high valuation of health and the enhancing of health should be borne in mind in all more specialised ethical discussions about health care. Such discussions often pinpoint certain problems in the enterprise. These problems must then always be balanced by a general utilitarian motivation for work towards health.

An Ethical Analysis of the Specific Categories of Health Promotion

With the help of the theoretical framework sketched on the preceding pages I shall now try to map some of the most important ethical problems in the field of health promotion.

I confine myself to ethical problems which deal with interaction between at least two agents, i.e. where there is a health-promoting agent and at least one recipient of this action, and where these two are distinct persons.

Let me first comment briefly on the direct kind of health promotion, i.e. the kind that involves direct manipulation of a person's body or psyche. This is the form of health promotion which most resembles standard health care and which is normally performed within the framework of institutional health care.

In cases such as these we can apply traditional health care ethics, which has been codified within ethical codes. We must then, in general, presuppose that the patient has voluntarily approached some health care institution in order to have a preventive measure performed. The doctor or some other member of the health personnel then performs this preventive action, if he or she considers it to be a measure *lege artis*. The action is performed in accordance with the generally accepted rule of complete informed consent. Respect for the patient's privacy as well as respect for the requirement of confidentiality is maintained with the same rigour as in traditional health care.

(Observe that I have not counted the directly manipulative kind of health promotion as an interaction. From an ethical point of view it is important, however, to remember that this kind of health promotion *presupposes* interaction in the form of communication between doctor and patient. It therefore presupposes ethical judgements on the part of the caring personnel. In particular, a directly manipulative treatment should never be forced upon a patient.)

But let us now scrutinise more closely the indirect kinds of interaction where we can make use of the practical syllogism. Let us start with a reasonably unproblematic case, i.e. one concerning component 4 in the syllogism, enabling or giving a person the opportunity to perform a health-promotive action.

Assume that the city of Linköping builds a sports centre for its inhabitants. Through this the population is given the opportunity to indulge in various kinds of sports in a more systematic and intense way than it could before. We presuppose here also that the sports in question are relatively harmless. (We exclude for the moment boxing and motor sports.)

Let us also assume that the city officials confine themselves to advertising this sports centre (i.e. they influence component 2 in the syllogism). They do not have influence in any other way. Can we find any ethical problems here? It is hard to see any. As long as the officials do not at the same time prevent the distribution of information about other possibilities of spending one's leisure time there has not been any limitation of the freedom of the inhabitants. The only thing that has happened is that the officials have provided more alternatives for people's lives. This form of health promotion is therefore quite unproblematic.

Now assume instead that the advertisement about the sports centre is supplemented with a recommendation to participate in the activities that are now provided. This recommendation can explicitly refer to the goal of health, for instance through the statement: if you wish to improve your health in a lasting way, then join in our new activities in the sports centre. In this case we have the salient influence (or creation) of component 3 in their practical syllogism on the part of those who already have the intention to maintain or restore their health.

The recommendation, however, need not refer to the goal of health. It can instead refer to some other goal assumed to be prevalent in the population. Suppose instead that the city officials say: if you want to make new friends then join in our activities; *or* if you want a beautiful body, then join our gang. If this type of recommendation turns out to be effective, then the syllogism that operates is something quite different, namely:

1. *A* intends to build up a beautiful body.
2. *A* has been informed about the sports centre and its activities.
3. *A* judges that given the new situation he will reach his goal of building up a beautiful body in the most efficient way if he uses the facilities of the sports centre.
4. *A* has the ability and opportunity to do this.

The activity which results from this syllogism will, if the initial health-promotive causal analysis is correct, also have the result that *A* enhances his health. That will then be an *unintended* consequence on the part of *A* but not on the part of the city official, who advertised for the sake of health promotion.

In these circumstances we have the seed of an ethical problem. Is it ethically defensible for a health promoter to conceal his or her main intentions and instead underline other consequences of a certain action, because he or she believes that the recommendation will be more effective if these consequences are highlighted? There are strong reasons for considering this question. One reason is that some evaluations of health-promoting campaigns, for instance, those performed by the Health Education Board for Scotland[5] have shown that messages which appeal to the interests of a particular audience can be much more effective, from the point of view of the health goal, than a standard informative message. The results indicate that, by imitating the techniques of the business marketeer, who very often appeals to people's strong longing for social and, in particular, sexual success, one can more effectively make people change their life-styles than by using the methods of traditional education.

Is this way of operating, in general, unethical then? And if so, why is it unethical? If we consider the case from a traditional medical ethical point of view we have a breach of the following ethical principle: a measure within health care shall be preceded by *adequate information* about the measure, about its purpose and its probable consequence. If, as in this case, a responsible city official (within a health-promoting office) issues a recommendation, it seems remarkable that there is no indication of the true purpose of the recommendation. A requirement of adequate information must follow from the general ethical codes of health care (a breach of the principle of informed consent is normally called *paternalism*).[6,7]

On the other hand it cannot generally be unethical to highlight the fact that there are further beneficial consequences (besides the health-promotive ones) of a proposed activity. To inform about this must be considered a supplementary contribution to the quality of a person's life. Yet again, one must pay ethical attention to the selection of further goals. Most people potentially have destructive drives and wishes. They can set up goals for their lives which are counter-productive in the long run. And it cannot be defensible to refer to such goals in the name of health care or health promotion.

Now consider attempts to influence component 1 in the syllogism, namely the direction of the will of the individual. We consider here those individuals who do not care about their health, and who do not consciously have a standing intention to protect their health. A diligent health promoter certainly is interested in influencing this category of people. How does such influence proceed?

This is a deep and difficult question. The question of what I call a *primary* influence on a person's will can hardly be rationally analysed. (By primary influence I mean an influence which is not based on a previously existing will on the part of the person to be influenced.) On the other hand there is a reasonable and very realistic *secondary* influence, which covers most of the relevant cases. The logic of such influence is the following. The starting point is to identify a goal that a person or a set of people in fact has. Imagine a student who wants to take a certain examination. Imagine further that he is in a difficult personal situation which is partly due to his bad health. If we want to help the student with his examination we ought to make him aware of the destructive influence that his low degree of health has on his work. We therefore tell him: if you wish to take your examination at the first opportunity, you must improve your health. If the student believes that our causal analysis is correct and still maintains his intention to take the examination, then for logical reasons he must also intend to raise his level of health. Thus, in a secondary way, he has formed the intention to raise his level of health.

What ethical aspects does this kind of case have? Normally it ought to be unproblematic. The goal of the subject has been taken seriously. What the health promoter does is to show that a high degree of health is a necessary condition for the realisation of the fundamental goal. The goal of health promotion coincides here in a happy way with the person's own primary goal.

From Health Education to Health Protection

Let me now treat a kind of interaction that is more common when we deal with societal or, in general, institutional measures. Primarily, I have in mind the measures of *legislation* and *price policy*. I thereby leave what is often called *health education* and proceed to *health protection*.[8] I shall first sketch an example.

The personnel at a government office have previously had great liberties concerning smoking and alcohol consumption at work. Following a ruling this behaviour is suddenly completely forbidden. As a result the behaviour of the personnel is changed drastically. They smoke and drink much less and their general state of health is gradually improved.

What character does this kind of interaction have? And which ethical aspects should be paid attention to?

The interaction in this case is, in an interesting way, different from that in the standard cases of health education. The practical syllogism which (normally) operates in this case of legislation has a very special intentional component (i.e. component 1). The legislator trusts that most citizens are law-abiding, i.e. have a standing intention to follow the laws and rules laid down in society. Then, if legislation is effective, the practical syllogism will have the following structure:

1. *A* intends to abide by laws and rules issued by the government.
2. *A* is informed about the new rules about drinking and smoking at government working places.
3. *A* understands that he can realise his standing intention only if he abides by this new rule.
4. *A* is capable of and not prevented from doing so.

Health promotion in the form of prohibition thus does not appeal to the citizen's own desires concerning health. In this respect price policy works in a similar way. Here the operating intention does not deal with laws, however. It concerns the individual's wish to protect his or her financial position. The individual acts according to the health promoter's will if he or she finds that a bottle of schnapps is too dear and abstains from buying such a bottle or at least buys fewer than before.

Measures of the above kind are more ethically controversial than most other measures. Why? The answer is that the citizen's actions are here influenced by a greater or lesser degree of *compulsion*. The citizen can no longer live the same way as before. The person's own value hierarchy no longer determines his or her life to the same extent. There is a restriction of autonomy.

What is compulsion? In previous texts I have analysed the case of an action performed under compulsion in the following way: a circumstance is compulsive for an agent to perform a particular act, if the circumstance seriously threatens the realisation of an intention that the agent is not prepared to give up.[9] A pistol threat is compulsive for every person who has the non-negotiable intention to survive. If one wishes, at any cost, to survive, then there is no alternative but to obey the gunman who threatens one with a gun.

So far I have only suggested a neutral characteristic of the notion of compulsion. I have not tried to judge its general ethical status. (I have no difficulty, however, in ethically judging the above example.) In fact, compulsion does not have a general ethical status. I think we see intuitively that there are cases of *justified* compulsion as well as of *unjustified* compulsion.

On an abstract plane I can provide two paradigm cases of justified compulsion. One case concerns such restriction of a person's freedom as to prevent the person from restricting someone else's freedom. The other is the case of force in preventing a person from severely hurting another person.

Our example with the prohibition from smoking in public buildings is a good example of a justifiable kind of legislation. The motivation for the prohibition has two facets. On the one hand it concerns the health of the smoker. On the other hand it concerns the health of the people surrounding the smoker. If a smoker is not conscious of the danger to the health of the surrounding population (or for that matter conscious of the general unease created by smoke), and is not prepared to pay respect to this, then we have a clear case of justified compulsion. However, it is not clear that it is equally justified to restrict the lonely smoker, i.e. to prevent him or her from smoking in a special room to which only smokers have access. A case of prohibition here might be a case of unjustified *paternalism*.

But have we now exhausted the cases of justified compulsion in the name of health? I shall make some further important additions. The cases to be discussed here all have to do with special characteristics of the recipient of the compelling action.

Consider first those people who have severe difficulty in understanding, or for whom it is impossible to understand, a health-promotive message. Typical examples of this are small children, senile people and some mentally handicapped people. If one wishes to influence these kinds of people it is rarely sufficient just to inform them about dangers to health, for instance about the dangers of their life-styles. In some cases the recipient clearly does not understand the message. In others it is unclear to what extent he or she understands it.

A health promoter who wishes to guarantee results with children, the senile and the mentally handicapped therefore often takes more drastic measures, like locking up things which he or she considers dangerous or deleterious, such as sweets, cigarettes or liquor. The people are then forcefully prevented from performing the (alleged) dangerous actions.

Is this kind of cumpulsion at all justified? I think that these cases deserve detailed scrutiny in all their instances. Perhaps I dare give some general comments.

The case with children is special in that the utility argument for health promotion is particularly strong in their case. One wishes to help them reach a platform of such health and intellectual maturity as can enable them to set autonomous goals and make autonomous choices in the future. Under these circumstances the utility argument is compatible with an argument from autonomy.

Children are different from the senile and the mentally handicapped in the sense that they are potentially autonomous. It must be our duty to help them become autonomous. A precondition for this is a minimal state of health during their development. Thus, a certain degree of compulsion is justified. The particular means of compulsion to be used ought to be selected with great care, however. Certain means, such as threat of physical or mental punishment, will probably be counter-productive for other reasons.

Active and compulsive health promotion directed towards the senile and the mentally handicapped has to be balanced against other utility arguments as well as arguments which have to do with the dignity of a human being. A first important point has to do with the age of the person. To work aggressively for the health of a very old person can lower this person's already low degree of quality of life. If there is no basic health to build upon then the pleasure of the moment can be well worth promoting.

So far I have offered some ethical points of view concerning those people who for intellectual reasons cannot absorb health education or other non-compulsive health promotion. But there is another important category that can motivate compelling measures for the sake of health. I have in mind those who understand the message very well but who cannot for other reasons change their style of life. Here we have two important sub-categories. The first consists of those who for social or other external reasons lack the ability to change their lives—perhaps the person lives in a very homogeneous and strong social environment which hardly permits divergencies in terms of food or other aspects of life-style.

A quite different sub-category consists of those who are forced by some *inner compulsion* to act in a certain, often destructive, direction. The most obvious cases are drug addicts who cannot be influenced by rational argument. To this category we can add all those cases of people with bad habits which are more or less difficult to break.

In both cases there is a lot of work to be done in the name of health but also in the general name of liberty and autonomy. Much of this work is so difficult as to require such extraordinary measures as are not traditionally counted as the business of health care. The matter of general social change is a political question and cannot be confined to the jurisdiction of a board of health promotion. On the other hand it is, of course, necessary for such a board to have a deep insight into the political and social conditions for health.

It is, for instance, essential to understand the importance of a culture for the course of people's lives, in particular when the culture is deeply rooted in religion. For instance, the life-style in an Islamic country is in many ways so culturally determined that only the strongest individualists can break away and create their own lives. If there were anything in the Islamic life-style (observe that this is hypothetical reasoning) that would be dangerous to people's health, then it would be virtually impossible just to approach an individual and suggest a change. The only practicable—and indeed the only really ethical—alternative would be to negotiate with the most senior and influential representatives of this religious culture.

It is easy to pinpoint obviously destructive life-styles within *subcultures* of our own Western societies. These can also involve strong elements of social compulsion, connected with threats of sanction if a particular person tries to leave the group. This is particularly so with some adolescent cultures in big cities who are often so welded together that a single individual can have enormous difficulty in leaving the community and breaking away from a life which perhaps involves criminality and drug addiction.

If criminality is involved, the ethical aspect becomes quite clear. Then we must be permitted to use force to prevent this way of living. Moreover, if children are involved the general argument about the protection of youth, which was used above, must be applicable. Otherwise, the ethical ground for *compulsory* intervention is much weaker. The case where the individual tries to break out and society comes in to help him or her is, of course, quite different and ethically easier.

Let me then proceed to discuss the phenomenon of *inner compulsion*. What is this and can it be characterised within the model of the practical syllogism? I believe that at least some types of this phenomenon can be clarified within the model. I particularly have in mind the case where we say that a person is determined by his or her *drives*. I shall develop my reasoning in the following way.

There are two things which have a central place in such action determination. First, every unsatisfied drive contains an element of unease. Second, the agent almost always knows from experience what the satisfaction of the drive means in terms of pleasure and ease.

Most people have a *prima facie* intention to satisfy an experienced drive, for instance the drives of thirst and hunger. The sensation of hunger thus functions as a reason for its bearer to take such action as will eliminate the sensation and thereby satisfy the drive.

Now our normal basic drives, such as hunger, thirst and sexuality, do not (except in very particular cases) involve health problems. Some acquired drives, however, in particular the ones involving drugs, are serious threats to the bearer's health. They also have the character of being immediately compelling. The agent feels a compulsion to have more of the drug.

The compulsion involved here can be clarified in the way proposed above. The addict considers the sensation of abstinence to be unbearable. The sensation is such that he or she is prepared to do anything to get rid of it. Given the situation, and indeed given the addict's general knowledge of the matter, he or she thinks that the intolerable sensation cannot be got rid of without more of the drug.

What ethical conclusions can be drawn from such a case of inner compulsion? Can they, in their turn, legitimate health-promoting actions of a compelling nature? For the ethical discussion there is a crucial difference between the categories of external and inner compulsion. External factors can often be removed without necessarily coming close to the person. But in order to remove a factor which constitutes or determines inner compulsion one must of necessity come very close to the person. The health-enhancing action may indeed involve medical treatment, and then the risk of violation of the person's integrity is much greater.

Now the ethical decision-making can be facilitated by the fact that most addicts are not always under the pressure of their drives and do not always suffer from the unbearable sensation of abstention. During such periods there is a case for rational discussion with them, and in particular for discussion about future strategies for action. The addict may then give permission to some other person to intervene by force and try to give treatment even in the face of the addict's own protests and apparent refusal.

It is much more problematic when a person is not conscious of his or her drive and does not consider it as being compelling, as in some cases of mental illness, for instance kleptomania and pyromania. Then it is more difficult to analyse the situation as compelling in my action–theoretical terms. However, this type of case falls outside the scope of this paper since it clearly comes within purely medical care, which was excluded from my initial definition of health problems.

Concluding Remarks

In this chapter I have tried to characterise the ethics of health promotion on the basis of a particular action–theoretical analysis. Such an analysis in fact also serves a basic theoretical and scientific purpose. Research on health promotion needs to structure its object. We have to clarify the borders of health promotion and identify its sub-categories.

For the action–theoretical platform I have been inspired by Professor von Wright's theory of action explanation. I have extended the application of this theory to the analysis of interaction between agents and to the general analysis of action determination. I have tried to show that this theory can classify effectively certain types of interactive actions within health promotion. It seems to me that this analytical tool is superior to the so-called health-belief model for health behaviour.[10]

An important fundamental in the study of health promotion is, of course, also the concept of health which is presupposed. If health is identified as the absence of disease, then health promotion will have a rather limited meaning. If health is positively defined as in this study, in terms of a person's ability to act in relation to his or her own goals then health promotion can entail something quite different.

The conceptual platform thus constructed can serve not only theoretical but also practical and ethical purposes. I have tried to use the system for a preliminary analysis of certain ethical problems within health promotion.

In particular I have noted various types of paternalistic behaviour, above all such paternalistic behaviour that entails *compulsion*. Both the concepts of paternalism in general and compulsion in particular have been analysed within the framework of the presented theory of action. It is my general conclusion that these kinds of action are the most problematic categories of health promotion. As a rule of thumb we should caution against paternalistic actions, in particular those which have a compulsory nature. But as I have also tried to argue there is an important category of *justified* paternalism which is required for the sake of health promotion.

References

1. Nordenfelt, L. (1987). *On the Nature of Health*, D. Reidel, Dordrecht.
2. Nordenfelt, L. (1991). *Towards a Theory of Health Promotion*, Linköping Collaborating Centre for WHO programmes, Health Service Studies 5, Linköping.
3. Wright, G.H. von (1971). *Explanation and Understanding*, Routledge and Kegan Paul, London.
4. Nordenfelt, L. (1974). *Explanation of Human Actions*, Dissertation, University of Uppsala.
5. Hastings, G. and Haywood, A. (1991). Social marketing and communication in health promotion. *Health Promotion International*, 6(2), 135–145.
6. Van de Veer, D. (1986). *Paternalistic Intervention*, Princeton University Press, Princeton.
7. Häyry, H.F. (1990). *Autonomy, and the Limits of Medical Paternalism*, Dissertation, University of Helsinki.
8. Downie, R.S., Fyfe, C. and Tannahill, A. (1990). *Health Promotion*, Oxford University Press, Oxford.
9. Nordenfelt, L. (1992). *On Crime, Punishment and Psychiatric Care*, Almqvist and Wiksell, Stockholm.
10. Rosenstock, I.M. (1990). The health belief model: explaining behavior through expectancies. In, *Health Behavior and Health Education: Theory, Research and Practice* ed. by K. Glanz, F.M. Lewis and B.K. Rimer, Jossey-Bass, Oxford.

Chapter 16

The Borders of Health Promotion

Alan Cribb

Centre for Educational Studies, King's College London, UK

Introduction

It is notoriously difficult to pin down the idea of health promotion. Indeed, it is even difficult to know what to call it, apart from an idea: is it an activity or a process, is it something we do or is it something that happens? Part of the peculiarity of calling it an activity is that is sounds so vague. If I leave the house in the morning saying, 'I'm just off to do some health promotion' it is far from clear what I'm going to get up to during the day. But the same might be said about other activities such as marketing. We would not usually describe our particular actions as marketing—we would talk about research, advertising, packaging, and pricing, etc. Marketing refers to a family of activities, each of which can be broken down further into particular actions. Perhaps health promotion is like this, and it does seem to be a helpful analogy, but we run into serious problems in identifying an equivalent family of activities. The set of activities appears almost boundless. In one sense it seems that health promotion is something that 'goes on' all the time, whether we are thinking about it or not, whether we are 'doing' it or not. Whatever our conception of health all kinds of activities and processes can be seen as promoting health. In this sense health promoting is like 'oxygen using'. All kinds of actions can be described as oxygen using, and so can various natural processes such as burning. Of course, the difference is that we would not talk of oxygen using as an activity in itself, as something we deliberately set out to do, as an occupation or profession, and so it is easier to live with its open-endedness.

This problem about the meaning of health promotion is of immense importance. It affects the way in which we think about the scope and priorities

Reforming Health Care: The Philosophy and Practice of International Health Reform.
Edited by D. Seedhouse. © 1995 John Wiley & Sons Ltd.

of health promotion, and it is integral to what I will describe, in the latter part of this chapter, as its central moral and political dilemma.

Nordenfelt's Analysis

In the previous chapter Lennart Nordenfelt has presented a systematic philosophical analysis of health promotion as a species of action. This analysis is very useful for understanding the nature of health promotion activities and evaluating them ethically. I want to raise some concerns about one element of this account. According to Nordenfelt's analysis, health promotion refers to that set of actions that are performed with the intention of maintaining or improving at least one person's state of health. Here it is the *intention*, and not the effect, that is the defining characteristic. I shall call this the 'intention condition'. Nordenfelt stresses this further by explaining, 'that there is no requirement that the action shall be effective with respect to health for it to be called a health-promotive action'.

I wish to look at two difficulties which attach to the intention condition. First, I look at the extent to which this condition is useful in an account of health promotion. Second, I consider the ambiguity of the condition. Initially I deliberately work with a narrow conception of health (where health means something like physical fitness and functioning)—even though this is narrower than Nordenfelt's conception. Later I consider some of the additional complications of working with a broader conception such as Nordenfelt's.

The Usefulness of the Intention Condition

Note that in the above quote Nordenfelt uses the expression 'be effective with respect to health' rather than 'maintain or improve health' or 'promote health', although he clearly means the latter. Perhaps this is to avoid the oddity of talking about health-promotive actions that do not promote health. Equally we might be reminded of actions that do promote health but which do not meet the 'intention condition' and are therefore not 'health-promotive actions'.

In order to discuss this I distinguish between things which are 'health causing' and things which are 'health pursuing'. Events, processes and actions can be health causing, but only actions can be health pursuing. An action is health pursuing if it is performed with the intention of pursuing health. Actions can be health causing without being health pursuing and vice versa. Thus if I walk to work to save my bus fare I am exercising, even if it is not my intention to 'take exercise', my action may be health causing even if it is not health pursuing. If one day I change my intention from saving money to taking exercise, the action becomes health pursuing but it does not necessarily become any more or less health causing. If we are interested in health promotion we must consider the whole domain of the health causing and not just the domain of the health pursuing. Nordenfelt limits 'health promotion' to the latter, it is all of those actions that take place in the pursuit of health.

This is a useful conception for certain purposes, in particular it fits the need of those people who see health promotion as their profession, or at least as a substantial part of their occupation or role. But it seems to me there are dangers in emphasising the intention condition. To put it in very general terms (so general that it may sound like a Zen-inspired paradox!)—the promotion of health is not necessarily best served by the pursuit of health. At a concrete level this means, for example, that a society in which people intentionally 'take exercise' is not necessarily one in which people get the most exercise (indeed the 'exercise life-style' is arguably the product of the sedentary life-style). Similarly, I will argue later that there are ways in which a health policy that is preoccupied with 'health gain' may be counter-productive. A fuller account of this depends upon some consideration of the meaning of 'health'. But first I want to return to Nordenfelt's taxonomy of health promotion.

His concentration on action and interaction is essential given his objective of placing health promotion in an 'action–theoretical context'. The overall analysis of the way different types of health promotion affects different components of action, and thereby raises different sorts of ethical issues is original and illuminating. Yet I am concerned that the concentration on action, interaction and the intention condition is misleading in a number of respects. The distinction I have made between health causing and health pursuing actions serves to illuminate what I regard as the peculiarity of some of Nordenfelt's examples. According to Nordenfelt a football match is 'health-promotive' if one of the players has a health-promotive purpose. If this player is substituted does the match cease to be health-promotive, or can the player's intention keep it health-promotive from the substitute's bench? Again, according to Nordenfelt, the building of a sports centre can be (indirectly) health-promotive if it is provided with the intention of improving health. Suppose we do not know the intention of the builders, must we be agnostic about whether to see it as part of health promotion? Surely if we wish to promote health what matters first and foremost, in this case, is that football is played and that sport centres are built, and the intentions of the footballers and builders is a secondary matter. It is normal to think of health promotion in terms of the consequences or effects of actions rather than, or as well as, their intentions.

The ethical issues which Nordenfelt considers mainly relate to what he defines as 'interactive health promotion':

> By interactive health promotion I mean here the case where an agent A influences another agent B to perform a directly health-promotive action.

This definition requires that B performs a health pursuing action rather than merely a health causing one (this is not because of the word 'directly' but simply a result of the intention condition). Yet the examples Nordenfelt gives encompass both cases. If B starts with an intention of maintaining or improving her health, or if A helps her form such an intention, then the health promotion is interactive in the above sense. But one type of health education and all the types of health protection that Nordenfelt discusses trade upon B's other intentions or purposes such as being beautiful, or obeying the law, or saving money. These examples do not conform to the above definition unless we ignore the intention condition. Also the distinction here between education and protection rests upon the differences between the medium of interaction (information versus legal/fiscal policy), whereas it might be argued that the term *health* education ought to be confined to only those cases in which the aim is to support (or bring about) B's intention to be healthy. As Nordenfelt argues, the other forms of interactive health promotion are more controversial from an ethical standpoint. They are more controversial precisely because the object is to get B to engage in health causing rather than health pursuing actions, either by manipulation or by compulsion.

The Ambiguity of the Intention Condition

Until now I have assumed that the intention condition is relatively clear, i.e. that it is fairly easy to tell whether or not it has been met with regards to a particular action. I do not think that this is the case. It seems that there are three possible readings:

1. *A* promotes *B*'s health where *A* thinks explicitly about improving or maintaining *B*'s health; that is where the idea of health forms part of the intention.
2. *A* promotes *B*'s health where *A* thinks about benefiting *B* in some way which is implicit in *A*'s conception of health.
3. *A* promotes *B*'s health where *A* thinks about benefiting *B* in some way which is implicit in *some* conception of health (for example, *B*'s conception, or some 'expert' or philosophical conception).

I will not analyse these possibilities fully but briefly discuss the alternative readings, and attempt to illustrate the practical importance of the ambiguity. Reading 1 seems too restrictive, it does not seem necessary to think in terms of health to be engaged in deliberate health promotion. If *A* has the intention of increasing *B*'s physical fitness or stamina it would seem absurd to deny that this is deliberate health promotion. Health and fitness are sufficiently closely related ideas for us to say the intention condition is met. Here we would expect that, if asked, *A* would connect these two ideas together, and this is the strength of reading 2. Even if *A* does not think explicitly about health in relation to the action, we can assume that *A* is operating with some (perhaps unconscious) conception of health which is related to and does inform the action. Reading 3 seems too open-ended. It seems wrong to say that *A* can have an intention to promote health unless what he is doing is closely linked to his own conception of health. Nordenfelt's examples of health promotion do not make it necessary to make a distinction between reading 2 and reading 3, because all of them relate to things which might reasonably be supposed to be part of most conceptions of health. However, if we insert Nordenfelt's broad conception of health into reading 3 the differences between 2 and 3 become very substantial, and we can no longer be neutral between the two readings.

Both readings generate problems. If we take reading 3 (with Nordenfelt's conception of health as the ability to realise vital goals) then all kinds of 'intentions to benefit' can be viewed as 'health promoting intentions', even when it would never occur to the agents that they were promoting health, or even when they might deny it. Thus teachers of English could be seen as operating with 'health promotion intentions', although they may personally deny having any such intentions, given their own conception of health. If we take reading 2 we make the ascription of 'health promotion intentions' dependent upon the agent's own conception of health. This means that A and B may act with broadly the same intention to benefit C in the same respect, and A has 'health promotion intentions' and B not. Despite this difficulty it seems that reading 2 is the most plausible and defensible reading of Nordenfelt's intention condition.

The Borders of Health Promotion

Taken together, these difficulties with the intention condition point to a deep ambiguity in Nordenfelt's chapter, and it is an ambiguity with important policy implications. Two conflicting pictures of the borders of health promotion are implicit in the chapter. One picture is implicit in the idea of 'health promotion intentions' and a different picture is implicit in Nordenfelt's conception of health. The former equates health promotion with whatever is done with 'health promotion intentions', that is roughly whatever is done in the name of health promotion. The latter equates health promotion with whatever actually promotes (maintains or improves) health (the ability to realise vital goals). The former, unlike the latter, is a hostage to whatever the prevailing conceptions of health happen to be. These two pictures of health promotion are manifestly different, and it is not difficult to imagine cases where they come into conflict. The obvious cases are those in which the would-be promoters are simply mistaken in their beliefs about what is of benefit. Although this sort of case is not of great philosophical importance it is clearly of great practical importance to the supposed beneficiary! The more subtle cases are those in which the intended benefit is real but in some way falls short of meeting, or even undermines, the overall 'health' of the intended beneficiary. It is impossible to discuss this further without making some summary remarks about the meaning of health.

Since the mid-1980s there have been a number of attempts to articulate what might be called a 'middle range' conception of health.[1-3] Before this the debate had largely been between a 'negative' disease-centred conception and a 'positive' well-being conception; the medical model versus the classic World Health Organisation (WHO) definition. The former can be seen as narrow but 'scientific', the latter as broad to the point of 'all inclusiveness', the challenge is to find an account somewhere in the middle. Although the newer middle-range accounts are significantly different from each other, and should be judged on their individual merits, they share some characteristics. They see health as a positive thing, something more than the absence of disease, but as something less than a state of complete well-being. Roughly speaking these accounts treat an individual's state of health as the degree to which an individual has the means to achieve well-being, in the sense of living 'a full life'. What is meant by a full life, and the degree to which a full life has to be 'one's own life', is one of the points of divergence between the accounts, and will not be discussed here. Health is the means to a full life; it is 'the foundations for achievement', or 'a resource for living', or 'the ability to realise vital goals'. For the purpose of this chapter I call this type of conception of health the 'welfare conception'. Welfare is a useful (if not exact) term here because it suggests ideas like 'having one's basic needs met' or 'enjoying some (specified) minimum level of well-being'.

As Nordenfelt argues, the welfare conception affects the borders of health promotion, because there are other elements to welfare (other necessary conditions for a full life) than disease-freedom. Yet in practice many of the things that go on in the name of health promotion are exclusively concerned with disease prevention. For example, health promotion is a key word in the UK government's *Health of the Nation* targets and policies.[4] But these are essentially about the prevention of death and diseases, not about the promotion of welfare or personal autonomy.

Health, however narrowly conceived, is connected to autonomy, because disease or disability act as constraints on autonomy. But under the welfare conception personal autonomy becomes a part of health, and the ideas of 'health promotion' and 'empowerment' become inextricably linked. This is most conspicuous in the WHO literature on health promotion[2,5] in which empowerment is arguably the central concept. I would argue that this literature relies on fudging together the two different pictures of health promotion. On the one hand, it trades upon the association between health promotion and disease management. Health promotion is what health care professionals do (or encourage others to do) in the name of health promotion; i.e. largely preventive medicine. In this context empowerment is the favoured process, the approved means to the end of health. On the other hand, the WHO literature suggests a broader view according to which empowerment is the end of health promotion, because autonomy is part of health. This latter view is not set out clearly and explicitly in the WHO literature, but I would argue that the literature is all the more influential because of this lack of clarity. The WHO literature and Nordenfelt's chapter suffer from the same ambiguity; the advantage of Nordenfelt's chapter is that it illustrates this ambiguity very sharply because he takes care to define his terms.

What is Healthy Public Policy?

The implications of the above ambiguity for policy are striking. Are we to set about minimising diseases or maximising welfare? Completely different perspectives and priorities are entailed by these alternatives. Only if we are clear about health can we interpret ideas like 'healthy public policy'. Philosophy, in its intolerance towards conceptual muddle, could be cast here as a useful servant of policy.

Yet if ambiguity is a weakness in philosophy it is sometimes a strength in politics. Health promotion can be seen as part of a political project to change cultures and social structures, including the direction and emphasis of public policy. In part this is an explicit project to 'reorient health services' and 'build a healthy public policy'.[5] Given these wholesale social and political goals the ambiguity of the term 'health promotion', and the confusion about its borders, is helpful. It is a term that brings together people of widely different interests and views. It draws much of its power from the neutral-sounding reference to 'health', which is an effective banner under which to mobilise people. It embraces those people who want to reduce the amount of disease in the world, including those who are professionally concerned with preventive medicine. Yet at the same time it is used as a term to contrast with preventive medicine—it is less 'medical', less 'disease-centred', more holistic, etc. Through its association with ideas like participation and empowerment it connects with those who have a more radical agenda. Finally, the broader interpretations of health as welfare, or even well-being, open a very wide agenda. Looked at in this way health promotion is a vehicle for transforming health care into social and political analysis and action, and it is a vehicle that works by associating together a lot of rather different, and sometimes conflicting, ideas.

I am not suggesting that exploiting the fuzzy boundaries of health promotion is a planned and collective strategy, rather that the development, use, and influence of the term owes a lot to its indeterminacy and rhetorical power. (To the extent that this is used as a strategy by individuals with a radical agenda it is likely to backfire, and there are signs of this happening in the UK. Just as health workers can get 'health promotion monies' for community action, the state can set 'health promotion targets' to regulate budgets. The rhetoric is sometimes based on a broad philosophy but the reality is nearly always defined by narrow models.)

As I have said, all discussions about health promotion policy or ethics depend upon an account of health. I am not trying to resolve this issue here, but I would like to look briefly at some of the methodological complications of working with a welfare conception rather than a disease conception of health.

Framing Interventions

If we consider a specific and direct intervention in preventive medicine, such as immunising a schoolchild, it is relatively easy to individuate and describe the characteristics of the intervention. From there we can start to make judgements about the merits of the intervention. It is aimed at a particular objective, it has certain risks or side-effects and so on. We can also ask whether the child made an 'informed choice', whether the parents or school authorities were properly consulted. As we reflect on these ethical questions the shape of the intervention becomes complicated. If the particular intervention is part of a programme, a whole population is affected by a set of policies. What are the value assumptions lying behind the policy and its organisation and delivery? Are the institutions and cultures of schooling being undermined or corrupted by using schools as the site for programmes of social regulation? In a few moments thought we have moved from the specific to the general.

If we want to consider specific disease-prevention interventions then we can draw an artificial frame around interventions. We can treat them as if they are independent of their social and policy context. Having framed the intervention it is still possible to raise meaningful evaluative and ethical issues—even though we may believe the wider policy and value questions to be more important. It could be argued that framing interventions in this way is morally and sociologically wrong-headed. Nonetheless it is possible to proceed in this way, indeed it is the approach taken by most traditional health care ethics.

However, it seems to me that this approach does not even make sense if we start from a welfare conception of health. Welfare is not promoted in an analogous way. It is possible to frame a relatively coherent set of 'disease-prevention intentions', but not an equivalent set of 'welfare-promotion intentions'. First, as was suggested above, things which might be framed as interventions are not typically aimed at welfare as such but are intended to produce a specific benefit. We grow vegetables, teach reading, build houses, but we do not normally 'promote welfare'. Second, to the extent that some of the things we do are welfare pursuing (rather than welfare causing) they pursue welfare indirectly, as a consequence of providing these other resources and skills. Again some interventions are self-consciously aimed at 'empowerment' but they are not aimed at empowerment in the abstract. Empowerment does not exist as an identifiable activity, or as the set of 'empowerment interventions'.

It is perfectly intelligible to talk about the promotion of welfare or autonomy providing we do not think that these describe domains of action in the same way that disease prevention does. We could follow an interest in the ethics of welfare promotion by identifying and framing some interventions, but it would be difficult to know where to start or how to frame them, and it would seem we were starting in the wrong place by missing out the wider processes and contexts. Whether or not a society provides its members with the means to a full life depends upon an analysis of the basic economic, social, cultural, and political forms of organisation—and only derivatively on the merits of specific interventions.

Nordenfelt concentrates on health pursuing actions because he is interested in health promotion as a deliberate activity. But the examples he uses all relate to a narrow sense of health (despite his broad definition) because this is the only sense in which health promotion as a domain of activity is meaningful.

The Central Dilemma of Health Promotion

How should we strike the balance between disease prevention and what I have called welfare promotion? I want to argue, at least for the purposes of this chapter, that this is the central ethical and policy challenge facing health promotion. It is easy to get bogged down in what might appear to be merely semantic issues. It could be argued that what I am calling welfare promotion just *is* health promotion. Others would say that health promotion should be more or less confined to disease prevention. Hence the terms in which the central dilemma is posed will vary according to who is speaking. Nevertheless it is a real dilemma for everyone. At its core is the value debate about the relative importance of living longer and less diseased lives compared to other conditions for 'the good life'. It is difficult to conceive of a policy or practical judgement that is not shaped by the positions we take in this debate. Attitudes towards the regulation of drugs or dangerous sports, palliative care or euthanasia, and more or less everything else turns upon it! The implications of the dilemma for health promotion policy can be summarised:

1. Strategies to prevent disease have other welfare costs and benefits (e.g. screening takes money from other goods and has psychological costs).
2. Much disease prevention is an indirect and unintended consequence of more general welfare promotion (e.g. transport and employment policies).
3. Therefore emphasis upon deliberate disease prevention risks (1) harming welfare overall and (2) harming disease prevention overall.

The WHO advocacy of health promotion is, in part, directed at this dilemma—we are to consider all of the determinants of health. We are to look at all of life through the lens of health promotion to make sure we optimise health. Unfortunately this only serves to aggravate the dilemma. For either we read health as the absence of disease, in which case we obscure the welfare costs and benefits; or we have a broader reading of health (such as the 'resource for living' suggestion) in which case we obscure the dilemma altogether.

I have deliberately confined my remarks to the tensions between a narrow conception of health and welfare, and not looked at the futher tensions between welfare and well-being which compound the ethical and policy problems. But things are already complicated enough. On the one hand there is good reason to aim for disease prevention particularly given the notorious inequalities in morbidity. On the other hand there are reasons to be wary of emphasising this as an aim. There are crucial ethical problems raised by this emphasis. But there are also methodological problems. An analysis that takes what is done 'in the name of health promotion' as its subject is likely, as Nordenfelt's does, to focus upon specific actions or interventions. This focus is not suited to capturing the wider processes of disease prevention. More important it is liable to obscure the possibilities and processes of empowerment.

References

1. Seedhouse, D. (1986). *Health: The Foundations for Achievement*. John Wiley and Sons, Chichester.
2. WHO (1986). A discussion document on the concept and principles of health promotion. *Health Promotion* **1**(1), 73–76.
3. Nordenfelt, L. (1987). *On the Nature of Health*. D. Reidel, Dordrecht.
4. Department of Health (1992). *The Health of the Nation*. HMSO, London.
5. WHO (1986). *Ottawa Charter for Health Promotion*. World Health Organisation and Health and Welfare, Ontario, Canada.

Chapter 17

Bad Faith and Victim-blaming: The Limits of Health Promotion

Charles J. Dougherty
Center for Health Policy and Ethics, Creighton University, Nebraska, USA

Behaviour and Health

The link between individual behaviour and health status is not a new discovery. Nor is the assignment of moral responsibility for behaviour that undermines health. The ancient Greeks believed that an individual was to blame if he became sick when preventing it was in his power. The Roman physician Galen thought people culpable for harms they had the knowledge and power to prevent. Medieval Europeans identified personal excess as a proximate cause of illness in many cases. However, the ancients also recognised the importance of heredity and social position in determining health status, and medievals finally referred illness and death to God's Will.[1]

In our times, tension between these two perspectives has increased. As the causal relationship between an individual's behaviour and disease becomes clearer, health promotion strategies that seek to educate and motivate individuals—and which thus implicitly or explicitly hold them accountable—appear more reasonable. On the other hand, the influence on health status of genetics, socio-economic position, and other factors beyond an individual's control are increasingly hard to deny. These latter considerations suggest aggregate and socio-economic strategies for health promotion, and tend to minimise or excuse the role played by individuals.

Should the individual, wholly or in part, be held responsible for his or her health? Or, should an individual's health be regarded as determined, wholly or largely, by factors outside the individual's control? Those who answer yes to the

Reforming Health Care: The Philosophy and Practice of International Health Reform.
Edited by D. Seedhouse. © 1995 John Wiley & Sons Ltd.

former question may be said to hold a *Freedom Model*; those agreeing to the latter, a *Facticity Model*.[2] The case for each of these models will be examined theoretically and with regard to strategies for health promotion. Finally, some thoughts will be offered on the development of a framework for health promotion that admits insights from both models.

Freedom and Bad Faith

The freedom model holds that the typical adult is capable of making a range of free choices that help to shape his or her life. Though no one can shape the facts that form the foundation of life—for instance, genetic inheritance, time and place of birth, initial socio-economic circumstances, and early childhood training—mature minors and adults make choices that continually shape their given circumstances into a life of their own. Of course, factors beyond an individual's control erupt throughout the course of all lives. But at the core of the freedom model is the belief that humans are capable of moments of reflection in which alternatives are surveyed and voluntary decisions are made. These are moments of self-determination and they can be found throughout the range of conscious experience, from the mundane choices of wardrobe and eating to the defining choices of mates and careers. The cumulative effect of such choices, intertwined with events that simply occur, is the creation of a person's life.

On this model, personal responsibility is located not only in choices that are consciously free, but also in those that are not but should have been. Thus a person can, for instance, be held responsible for ignoring or forgetting duties, for not having knowledge that he or she should have had, for being reckless or careless, or for the consequences of unchecked passions or addictions.

Human dignity is a central notion on this model. People have dignity, in part, because of their ability to make free choices and to be responsible for them. People are worthy of respect because of this creative potential, this ability to be self-determining. Since people can shape at least part of their destinies, they can be held responsible for what they do shape or fail to shape in their lives. We can take some credit and must also bear some blame for the lives that we lead.

Each of us has experienced the phenomena associated with a free choice—a sense of distancing from the normal pace of behaviour and events, the scrutinising of options and their consequences, the anguish of indecision, the feeling of release and conviction (sometimes burden) of having made a decision. We have all experienced as well the times in which the options for free choice seem to narrow under the pressures of circumstances, the demands of others, or the force of habits. Yet ambiguous experiences that are a mix of freedom and coercion do not obscure the basic polar reality that some choices and actions are voluntary and some are not. Some things I choose; some happen to me. Sometimes I am responsible; sometimes I am not.

Freedom and responsibility is routinely presumed both in self-evaluation and social interaction. In ordinary experience, those who deny freedom and responsibility are generally thought to be in bad faith, in a kind of knowing self-deception, for the sake of avoiding moral accountability.

The Freedom Model and Health Promotion

Among the compelling reasons for applying the freedom model to the challenges of contemporary health promotion is the amount of information now available that links individual behaviour with health status. It is increasingly clear that some choices, habits, and life-styles help to prevent disease while some help to create it. A 1979 US government report, *Healthy People*, estimated that 50% of mortality was due to life-style and unhealthy behaviour. The report noted a 21% decline in death from coronary heart disease in the US between 1968 and 1976 and linked the decline to better diet and reduced smoking. A follow-up report in 1990, *Healthy People 2000*, underscored the same point by linking major declines in the leading causes of death in the US in the 1980s to reductions in behaviour-related risk factors involving smoking, diet, control of hypertension, and automobile safety.[3]

The same point was made provocatively in 1977 by Dr John Knowles, then president of the Rockefeller Foundation. He argued that early 20th century advances in health status depended on public economic and environmental policies but that further advance in the late 20th century would be based directly on the behaviour and habits of individuals. Thus, he claimed, talk about a 'right' to health had to be replaced by individual responsibility to preserve one's own health and to control the public costs of 'sloth, gluttony, alcoholic intemperance, reckless driving, sexual frenzy, and smoking ...'[1] Knowles' words may strike the contemporary reader as overly judgemental, yet a 1990 study of the leading life-style risk factors among patients in a suburban family practice in the American midwest identified a similar list (excepting 'sexual frenzy'): smoking, excess alcohol use, obesity, sedentary life-style, lack of seat belt use, use of hazardous transportation vehicles and inadequate rest. Of these, the study found that the most prevalent adverse habits were lack of seat belt use (77% of the sample of 147 patients) followed by sedentary life-style (44% of the sample).[4]

It is also well known that life-style changes can have a positive impact on an individual's risk of chronic disease. Because multiple risk factors for a single individual can have a synergistic effect, the benefits of positive behaviour change are even greater for those at greatest risk from several unhealthy habits. Moreover, there can be significant psychological benefits to the individual from successful behaviour change: enhanced self-esteem, increased sense of self-control, reduced anxiety, increased energy, and greater ability to be calm and focused.[5]

Health benefits from changes of individual behaviour can be identified even in especially challenging areas. Preterm birth, for example, is a major health problem in the US, especially in the inner cities. It contributes to 60–80% of America's high perinatal mortality rate. A 1990 study of inner-city women in the US who were at high risk for preterm birth identified a number of life-style and stress factors that are implicated in preterm delivery. Not all of them are under any single individual's control, for example, longstanding financial difficulties and drug use by family members. But women at high risk who were able to decrease long work hours, heavy lifting, and sexual activity were more likely to deliver at term.[6] In general, the contemporary women's health movement has been telling women to 'take charge of their health', and has helped to highlight the life-style changes that can serve to avoid or minimise urinary incontinence (a leading cause of nursing home admission), osteoporosis, stroke, breast and lung cancer, and heart disease.[7]

Some of America's worst health statistics—among the urban minority populations with low socio-economic status—have proven impervious to large improvements through health promotion activities designed to generate voluntary changes in personal behaviour. But the connection between life-style and the major health deficits of these communities is clear. It is possible that socio-economic barriers to positive life-style change can be overcome when 'community-based organisations are mobilised to incorporate self-help, community empowerment, and health behaviour change as priorities . . .' in health education interventions.[8]

According to the freedom model the individual is morally obliged to try to make changes in habit and life-style that will promote better health status. This obligation can be grounded in two ways, as a duty to others and as a duty to self. The former is the easier case to make. Because individual life-style changes can be made—people do stop smoking, use seat belts, and moderate their alcohol consumption—then they should be made. The moral force of this conclusion comes from the premise that we are each obliged to avoid or minimise harm to others, and poor health and premature death generally do harm others. Such harm can include loss of ability to discharge responsibilities to spouses, family members and friends; reduced effectiveness at work and in other areas of social contribution, and the increased cost of health care that is distributed to others through insurance pools, welfare arrangements, or national health care programmes. This latter point has become a special contemporary concern as many nations are reaching fiscal and political limits in their health care spending, forcing them to make difficult allocation and rationing decisions.[9,10]

The basis for an obligation to try to be healthy is harder to identify when it is wholly self-referential. If my obligation to be healthy is to myself, then I can release myself from it whenever this obligation conflicts with another personal interest, in particular when it conflicts with the pleasures of unhealthy habits.[11] Thus a duty to oneself to try to be healthy appears to be a rather anaemic duty, perhaps no duty at all.

Yet, this analytical account does not do justice to the moral psychology that many experience. The ability to live a healthier life is associated with enhanced self-esteem while failure to make life-style changes can create the opposite effect.[6] One hypothesis that would explain this moral psychology is that people do sense what amounts to a duty to preserve or enhance their own health status. Therefore, they feel good about themselves when they discharge this duty and bad about themselves when they do not. The freedom model can admit a wide range of extenuating circumstances that weaken the degree of responsibility individuals bear in many cases.[12] What the freedom model cannot do, however, is deny the voluntary component of many health-related behaviours, including habits of smoking, eating, and drinking, as well as decisions to ski, sunbathe, and omit seat belts. To some degree, varying in individual cases, individuals are responsible for these behaviours. To hold otherwise is to renounce the central belief that persons—at least to an extent—are autonomous, and able to shape their own destinies.[13] And it weakens or destroys the grounds for belief in human dignity.

Facticity and Victim-blaming

On the facticity model human behaviour emerges from a nexus of facts over which no individual has control. Behaviour is caused not chosen, and so are the resulting conditions of health or disease. As a consequence, the assignment of responsibility to individuals who suffer from deteriorated health and premature death due to behaviours not of their own choosing is a form of blaming the victim, a second punishment with social disapproval of those who have already been punished by circumstances.

Perhaps the strongest element of the facticity model is the argument from genetics. Through no merit or blame on the individual's part, each of us inherits a genetic blueprint that determines large parts of our future: gender, race, ethnic group, general condition of health and general appearance. It is also plausible to believe that other important facts are strongly shaped by genetic inheritance: general intelligence, degree of susceptibility and resistance to certain diseases, and general psychological dispositions. Furthermore genetics may play a significant role in sexual orientation, addiction to alcohol and smoking, obesity, and other habits that have health implications.

Genetics, of course, only sets the stage for the myriad of other determining factors that shape an individual's life. Environmental factors surround the developing child and shape his or her emerging personality. The actions and dispositions of parents, other family members, and caretakers fix his or her immediate social world. That social world is itself determined by the socio-economic status of the family. And rules for behaviour, expectations for the future, and general world-view are formed by such factors as racial and ethnic identification, family income, degree of education, and stability of relationships.

By the time of maturity, an individual is thoroughly infused with the facts that have created his or her past. On the facticity account moments of reflection and choice, so stressed by the freedom model, are merely moments of intersection between perceptions of the present and competing influences from the past. The specific moment of choice vanishes upon subsequent reflection into the causes that led to it—the genetics, habits, and lifetime of other influences that brought the individual to that moment and determined the content of choice.

On the facticity model people are not free to be other than what they are. They *are* their roles, their habits, their inheritance. They are reflections of their genetics and the social and economic environment they inhabit. Responsibility is not appropriately placed on individuals but on the political, economic, and cultural systems that create the social context for their lives. To hold individuals who have already suffered because of the facts of their circumstances accountable for 'free' choices, is to blame people who are already victims.

What is fundamentally important to the facticity model and what gives life to the notion of human dignity is active sympathy with the struggles of others. Belief in human dignity requires sympathy with those trapped in conditions that stunt human development, and a commitment to social action to promote change in a positive direction. Sympathy and social action should be oriented to where the real levers of change exist—toward communities, politics, and the economy. By contrast a misplaced focus on the individual will lead away from the practical work of building better societies and toward romantic notions of self-improvement that inevitably set the stage for victim-blaming.

The Limits of Individual Control

In 1981 a US opinion poll reported that 51% of adults believed they had 'a great deal' of control over their future health; 36% more believed they had 'some control'. Another poll taken in 1986 found that 93% of Americans surveyed agreed that 'if I take the right actions, I can stay healthy'. Yet in an area that should display considerable evidence of individual control—dieting for the sake of health and a more attractive body—experience of control is slim. Despite widespread dissatisfaction with the body and an 'epidemic of dieting', the experience of many who have tried to diet is not of control but of repeated and frustrating cycles of weight loss and regain. One plausible account for this paradox is that while people believe they control their body size through diet, more of the variance in people's weight and shape—even where fat is distributed on the body—may be accounted for by genetics.[3]

Control also seems to be at issue in attempts to locate 'the' cause of a disease or premature death in the behaviour of an individual. But identifying 'the' cause of any human event is far more complex than it may appear initially. Every traffic-related death, for example, has multiple causes; a set of conditions is conjointly necessary for the accident to have occurred. In a given case these conditions might include the fact that the deceased wore no seat belt; that the road surface was slippery; that the evening was dark and the road poorly lit; that there was no traffic signal at the intersection; that the community refused to tax itself to create better rail or bus connections; that automobiles travel at high speed, stop slowly, and weigh hundreds of pounds; that human bodies are fragile; that there are laws of physics; that this was the Will of God; and so on. In spite of this spate of candidates for 'the' cause, people are inclined to choose as the cause of an untoward health event those factors perceived to be under the immediate control of the individual. We are more likely to lament the fact that the driver wore no seat belt than that automobiles are constructed as they are, in spite of the fact that both causes were necessary for the outcome.[12]

Women with high-risk pregnancies who are able to avoid long work hours, heavy lifting, and sexual activity increase their chances of delivering at term. But what shapes their ability to adopt these preventive measures? When a nation has no policy of work leave and income protection, many women with high-risk pregnancies simply cannot afford to leave work. Many low-paying jobs, including the non-paying jobs of housekeeping and home child care, inevitably involve both long hours and heavy lifting. And limiting sexual activity is not a decision all women can make for themselves.[7]

Even the influence of cigarette smoking during pregnancy on preterm birth is equivocal. The effects of maternal smoking on the fetus are often negligible when the woman belongs to the upper middle class, but are magnified by lower socio-economic status.[14] What then caused a particular instance of preterm birth—maternal smoking or maternal poverty? Suppose that maternal smoking is identified as the cause—again, it is proximate and appears to be under the individual's control. But what permits some smokers to quit and makes it nearly impossible for others to quit? In particular, what is the cause of this woman's continued smoking? It is known that smokers whose friends and family smoke are generally less likely to quit and that smoking prevalence has a marked socio-economic aspect—45% of blue collar Americans smoke and only 20% of professionals. So even if social facts are ignored at first and maternal smoking identified as the cause of a preterm birth, they can become the cause again. If the majority of this woman's friends and family smoke and all of them are at the lower end of the economic scale, then social facts caused her continued smoking which in turn caused the preterm birth.[6]

This point can be generalised. In addition to the clear link between socio-economic status and smoking, powerful economic and social forces shape the amount of exercise taken, drinking habits and diet. Diet, for example, is affected by local and ethnic customs, nature and amount of education, availability and price of foods, advertising, decisions by farmers, transporters and merchants, government policies, etc.[15] In some cases, poor diet and other high-risk behaviours may also provide an escape from the grim realities of poverty, expressing the despair produced by living conditions that offer no hope for a better future.[16]

Part of the explanation for the attractiveness of identifying the individual cause as 'the' cause is that such judgements are often made by people not facing the stresses of low socio-economic status about people who are. The moral logic goes something like this: (1) 'I stopped smoking'; (3) 'Therefore, she can stop smoking'. But suppressed in this enthymeme is the middle term needed to link the explicit premis to the conclusion. Logically, it would have to have the form: (2) 'She is able to do what I have done'. Certainly she is able to do much of what I have done; we are each human. But the conclusion that she can stop smoking does not follow if some of the differences in our social situations are spelled out. (1) 'I stopped smoking (with the support of my non-smoking family and professional friends, under the supervision of my family physician, with the help of temporary nicotine supplements paid for by my health insurance, and with a financial incentive from my white-collar employer)'; (2) 'She is (not) able to do what I have done (because she has none of these social supports)'; (3) 'Therefore, she can (not) stop smoking'.

Negative stereotypes about the poor compound the problem. A 1989 study of 240 nurses in the US—a group that might be expected to be sympathetic—found many negative attitudes towards the poor. Over half the sample (58%) believed that poor women become pregnant to collect welfare benefits and 43% agreed that poor people prefer to stay on welfare. To the claim that poverty is a result of lack of effort, there was 36% agreement; 27% agreed that poverty is due to squandered opportunities; and 43% agreed that the poor try to 'take advantage of' the health care system.[17]

All the ingredients for victim-blaming are now in place. Behaviour, including habits and life-style, are under an individual's control. His or her choice is 'the' cause of the behaviour and the resulting health consequences. No allowance is made for substantively different circumstances; everyone can make healthy choices. Therefore, people who do not make healthy choices have voluntary character flaws—laziness, dependency, exploitativeness. They do not deserve assistance; they deserve the poor health they choose through their own freedom. The victim of facts beyond his or her control is thus blamed for moral failure as well.

Part of this inclination to blame the victim may derive from a general psychological tendency to have negative feelings about people who are suffering or in need of help. The perception of vulnerability in others makes us feel vulnerable too and undermines belief in control.[3] When this victim-blaming attitude is conveyed by health care professionals caring for the vulnerable, it can actually worsen a patient's burden of suffering. A patient with acute cardiac disease, for example, experiences anxiety, fear, and loss of control from the disease itself. If he is aware that the aetiology of his disease in the minds of his doctor and nurses is his moral failure, his slothful life as a 'couch potato', this suffering can be compounded with feelings of responsibility, guilt, and remorse.[18] In spite of the fact that socio-economic status remains the best predictor of preterm birth, the mother who smoked may be blamed by the neonatology team for her baby's difficulties. Responsibility is shifted from society to the individual.[17] And there is no release from blame by appeal to the conditions of poverty, not if being in a state of poverty is itself considered evidence of moral failure.[17]

Freedom Without Victim-blaming; Facts Without Bad Faith

Understood as a problem of metaphysics, as the freedom versus determinism debate, there is little hope for resolution of the conflict between the freedom model and the facticity model. The history of Western philosophy is testament to the perennial character of this dispute.

But the issue at hand is not as thoroughly impassable. The freedom model does not hold that all human behaviour is free, not even all deliberate choice. Plainly, a great deal of behaviour is physically involuntary: autonomic bodily responses, the most basic attractions and repulsions, shoves in a crowd. Another layer of behaviour is so plainly conditioned by context as to be largely beyond most individuals' routine control: reactions of 'fight or flight', actions patterned by rules of social interaction, the historically and culturally determined world views of the age. Finally, even in the range of behaviour regarded as voluntary and under, or potentially under, an individual's control, the freedom model can recognise a vast array of excusing and mitigating conditions that blunt the assessment of responsibility and thus avoid the indictment of 'blaming the victim'. The core of the freedom model is that *some* human behaviour is free and *sometimes* attributing both praise and blame is appropriate and even necessary. The project of identifying voluntary behaviour and determining when to praise and blame is inherently practical and context-dependent.

There is room for movement in the facticity model as well. Although it may appear in some versions of this view that freedom itself is being denied, this is not so for all those who are concerned about blaming victims. In these cases, freedom and responsibility is not denied, rather its locus is shifted from the individual to society. Placing too much stress on individual control can lead to missed opportunities to confront environmental causes of disease.[3] The individual strategy is 'cheap' because it calls for no change in the social environment.[17] The proper locus for health promotion activities is the public policy process and community empowerment.[16] Political advocacy is called for: greater citizen participation in voting and lobbying, organising coalitions, and monitoring the effects of public programmes.[19]

Thus the facticity model is not rightfully charged with the bad faith that seeks exemption from all responsibility. Instead, a strong sense of political responsibility is asserted. In many cases, there is no shortage of blaming either. But instead of the victims of behaviour-related diseases, blame is placed on those thought to be responsible for the ills of society—the wealthy and well, politicians, indifferent citizens. Thus at least some individual freedom is asserted or conceded, namely, the freedom—and responsibility—of individuals to try to improve health by changing the socio-economic system. Assessment of the changes needed and the degree of responsibility of individuals for the system, and for changing the system, is also a practical and context-dependent task.

Therefore, though apparently irreconcilable in metaphysics, in the practical context of health promotion, 'openings' exist in each model. There is an admission of facticity—potentially a great deal of it—by the freedom model and an admission of some individual freedom by the facticity model. These openings allow for the possibility of developing a framework for health promotion that reconciles these competing views. Progress in this direction can be made by reconsidering the main insight of each model from a practical point of view. The questions to be asked are:

1. What is the central policy concern of each model, the chief fear that motivates it?
2. How can that concern be met most effectively in a scheme that also addresses the other model's greatest concern?

The central concern of the freedom model is the putative bad faith of avoiding individual responsibility for behaviour that appears to be under an individual's control. Theoretically, this denial of individual freedom and responsibility can undermine the important notion of human dignity. But the deeper practical concern seems to be the fear that failure to identify individual choice as the cause of behaviour-related diseases will lead to lack of individual effort, to a failure to try to keep oneself healthy and to try to restore health when it is lost. Such a result is considered to be harmful to the individuals involved and to society. It is thought to encourage or condone irresponsible behaviour on the part of individuals, thereby increasing bad health outcomes. It is also said to create social dependency: individuals become 'voluntary victims' by blaming the consequences of their own choices on others. It is further believed that lack of individual effort creates new costs for society by increasing the need for health care resources and by distributing these additional costs unfairly on those who have made efforts to be healthy.

The central concern of the facticity model is the victim-blaming that results when individuals are held accountable for health states that follow from their own behaviour. When individual choice is seen as 'the' cause, individuals already suffering from diseases and/or poor social conditions are made to suffer further from feelings of guilt and failure. The theoretical argument is that this is unjust since free choice is not a cause at all. But at a deeper practical level, the motivating fear of the facticity model seems to centre on the potential for loss of sympathy with those in need. Health promotion efforts that focus solely on individual behaviour promote stereotyping and the hardening of public attitudes toward the unhealthy. For example, a public advertising campaign that states explicitly that 'Responsible people control their blood pressure' or 'Mothers who care get prenatal care', also states implicitly that those who do not are irresponsible and uncaring. Moreover, the lack of sympathy which may be promoted by victim-blaming in the clinical setting can undermine the traditional altruism of health care.

A Policy Framework for Health Promotion

A health promotion framework that does justice to the main concern of each model, must, therefore, promote individual effort by all and maintain public sympathy for those in need. These goals can be met if the notion of cause is stratified as follows.

1. In health education efforts, the individual should be assumed to be 'the' cause. When people are given information about the health implications of various personal behaviours, the message must be that people *can* choose behaviours that lower risk and improve health. Not only does this seem to be the honest truth, it is also empowering. Compared with the alternatives of avoiding individual health education or freighting it with qualifiers about the social context, this approach makes direct appeal to the dignity of each individual. It addresses people as individuals with some say over their destinies. It denies that people are merely passive vehicles for their own habits and offers a degree of control and therefore of self-esteem. It asks individuals to make the effort, to try to stay healthy and to return to health when sick.

2. Health education efforts should generally be conducted in the context of overall health planning, in conjunction with a range of health promotion

efforts. In these efforts, the individual should be assumed to be only one cause of many causes and generally not the most important or useful cause to address. Focus here should be on the facts that mitigate or remove individual control over health-related behaviour. Efforts to eliminate harmful genetic traits, to create employment and improve housing to make automobiles safer and curb the use of guns—these are critically important in improving the general health of society. This approach plainly entails political efforts. It requires a community focus, consensus building, and the creation of public programmes. It also requires educational efforts to contain stereotyping of those who are unhealthy, especially those who are doubly vulnerable due to low socio-economic and/or minority status. In this context, respect for human dignity is expressed in efforts to improve the social facts that give context to the practical exercise of individual freedom.

3. Regardless of the success of programmes of health education and health promotion, people will get sick, people will still die. In these moments of need, there should be universal access to non-judgemental personal care. Individual choice should not be considered a cause at all in these clinical settings. If an aetiology must be offered, many other causes are readily available. There is no justification for choosing the one putative cause—individual choice—that is bound to cause additional suffering to patient and family. Counselling aimed to return a patient to health and to avoid future problems can identify behaviours that are mandatory or favourable or that must be minimised or avoided altogether. Such counselling can be done, however, without indicting the individual's past behaviour for the present health problem. This too is a matter of honesty. No behaviour or life-style is guaranteed to produce a particular disease; equally no behviour or life-style assures longevity.[18] Respect for human dignity in the clinical context means cultivating and preserving a sense of sympathy for the sufferings of fellow human beings, whether they are free or not.

Conclusion

This framework does not resolve all the tensions between the freedom model's concerns about bad faith and the facticity model's concerns about victim-blaming. It does provide a platform for a dialogue between two competing views of the person, views that may appear incompatible theoretically but views that can complement each other in the practical context of health promotion. The framework stratifies the notion of causation in the link between individual behaviour and health status. In this manner, health education can be used to encourage individual effort, health promotion activities can be designed to improve the social environment, and sympathy for the sick and poor can be protected in clinical encounters. There is a role in health promotion for a notion of individual freedom that does not foster victim-blaming and a respect for the power of facts that does not encourage bad faith.

References

1. Reiser, S.J. (1985). Responsibility for personal health: A historical perspective. *Journal of Medicine and Philosophy* **10**, 8–10.
2. Names for the models and some of the insights that follow are drawn from Sartre, J.P. (1956). *Being and Nothingness.* Philosophical Library, New York.
3. Brownell, K. (1991). Personal responsibility and control over our bodies: when expectations exceed reality. *Health Psychology* **10**(5), 303–310.
4. Chao, J. and Zyzanski, S. (1990). Prevalence of life-style risk factors in a family practice. *Preventive Medicine* **19**, 533–540.
5. Ockene, J., Sorensen, G., Kabat-Zinn, J., Ockene, I. and Donnelly, G. (1988). Benefits and costs of life-style change to reduce risk of chronic disease. *Preventive Medicine* **17**, 224–234.
6. Freda, M.C., Anderson, H., Damus, K., Poust, D., Brustman, L. and Merkatz, I. (1990). Life-style modification as an intervention for inner city women at high risk for preterm birth. *Journal of Advanced Nursing* **15**, 364–372.
7. Newman, D. (1987). Taking charge: A personal responsibility. *Public Health Reports Supplement* July/August, 74–77.
8. Thomas, S. (1990). Community health advocacy for racial and ethnic minorities in the United States: Issues and challenges for health education. *Health Education Quarterly* **17**(1), 18.
9. Hackler, C. (1993). Health care reform in the United States. *Health Care Analysis* **1**, 5–13.
10. Have, H.A.M.J. ten (1993). Choosing core health services in The Netherlands. *Health Care Analysis* **1**, 43–47.
11. Gorovitz, S. (1978). Health as an obligation. In, *Encyclopedia of Bioethics*, ed. by W. Reich, pp. 606–609. The Free Press; New York.
12. Dworkin, G. (1981). Taking risks, assessing responsibility. *Hastings Centre Report* **11**, 26–31.
13. Veatch, R. (1980). Voluntary risks to health. *Journal of the American Medical Association* **243**, 50–55.
14. Romita, P. and Hovelaque, F. (1987). Changing approaches in women's health: New insights and new pitfalls in prenatal preventive care. *International Journal of Health Services* **17**(2), 249.
15. Townsend, P. (1990). Individual or social responsibility for premature death? Current controversies in the British debate about health. *International Journal of Health Services* **20**(3), 383.
16. Mondragón, D. (1993). No more 'Let them eat admonitions': The Clinton administration's emerging approach to minority health. *Journal of Health Care for the Poor and Underserved* **4**(2), 80.
17. Price, J., Desmond, S. and Eoff, T. (1989). Nurses' perception regarding health care and the poor. *Psychological Reports* **65**, 1046–1048.
18. Marantz, P. (1990). Blaming the victim: The negative consequences of preventive medicine. *American Journal of Public Health* **80**(1), 1187.
19. McLeroy, K., Bibeau, D., Steckler, A. and Glanz, K. (1988). An ecological perspective on health promotion programs. *Health Education Quarterly* **15**(4), 366.

Chapter 18

The Purpose–Process Gap in Health Promotion

Ian Buchanan

Bury and Rochdale Health Authority, UK

Introduction

Health promotion is an eclectic profession which readily adopts methods developed by other disciplines (borrowing especially from medicine, education and psychology). This magpie-like tendency is so widespread that many health promotion theorists take it for granted that the processes and goals of the various parent disciplines have been successfully synthesised, and now form a unique and coherent whole: health promotion.

It is as if many different sets of activities (and sets of values) have been drawn to a health promotion temple to trade, whereupon they have been organised and marshalled by the controllers of the temple. The traders have been concerned to gain space in which to sell their wares, while the organisers (the health promotion theorists) have worked to establish broad ground rules for the operation as a whole. It has been assumed that the fact that trading is going on means that the various trades are co-existing in harmony, and that the temple is serving its proper purpose. But this is a highly questionable image.

Perhaps because the market has proved attractive to so many well-established traders there has seemed little need to discuss whether this is what ought to be going on in the temple. However, I believe that health promotion's traditional pattern of development—which has been to take a route from practice to theory—has placed far too much trust in *habit* and *opportunism*. Those practices which have happened to exist, or which have found a niche at a convenient time, have been allowed to define health promotion rationale. But clarity and unity can also come from the opposite direction (and indeed are far more likely to do so) that is, by attending to the question 'What, in the first place, is the end to which health promotion should be directed?'

Reforming Health Care: The Philosophy and Practice of International Health Reform.
Edited by D. Seedhouse. © 1995 John Wiley & Sons Ltd.

The Implicit Claims of the Health Promotion Movement

On the face of it the question 'to what end should health promotion be directed?' may appear impossibly nebulous, but in fact it is far from fanciful. Indeed by asserting its existence as a valuable enterprise health promotion already claims to have answered it.

In itself the term health promotion involves a series of implicit claims. Its use implies that the meaning of health is understood, that the activities undertaken as health promoting will create health according to this understanding, and that there is a demonstrable relationship between these activities and the promotion of health. By describing health promotion as a *movement* (as they frequently do), its advocates make the claim that a unified view of the direction and ends of health promotion exists, and is being followed. That is, it is claimed that the health promotion movement does not draw from a range of disciplines at *random*, but does so for a coherent set of reasons.

Purposes and Processes

If it is taken at all seriously health promotion must be able to *substantiate* its claims. Health promotion involves end-focused or purposive action. All health promotion activity is intended to improve a situation and its justification is dependent upon the nature of the intended improvement being known to the promoting agent. An important distinction can be made between purpose (end) and process (the means to an end). Purpose provides the definitional touchstone and the processes (the acts and activities, models, tools, techniques, approaches, systems, resources—human and other) which are applied to the achievement of purpose are of contingent significance only. The identity of health promotion purpose cannot therefore simply be determined by observing those activities purportedly undertaken in its pursuance. At some point the question of what it is that these activities seek commonly to do has to be satisfactorily addressed.

If no clear account of common purpose exists to illuminate how process contributions relate to its achievement, the success or failure of health promotion activities cannot be adequately tested (and the merits of the various processes cannot be meaningfully compared). Although most health promotion theorists offer 'process definitions', which focus primarily on activities and their taxonomy,[1,2] such definitions can be said to be substantial only if the purpose towards which they are directed is clear. Debate over process issues in health promotion has flourished over several years but any assessment of the constituent elements of the debate remains highly problematic. Some forms of synthesis are possible, but only on the basis of contingent compromise.

The 'Purpose Account' must be Achievable

It is important to note that health promotion is always said to be a practical discipline. It follows that whatever concept of health is said to encapsulate health promotion purpose, it will need to be a formulation that is achievable. If the 'health' of health promotion is chimeric, i.e. if the gap between process and purpose is allowed to extend beyond the possibility of practical achievement, then the basis of health promotion's essentially prescriptive claims is weak. An unambiguous and deliverable theory of health is required to confirm a strong case for health promotion.

A review of the literature in health studies reveals that a range of concepts exists. These various formulations, although they may be internally coherent, are not mutually compatible and they differ substantially with regard to the quality of the blueprint they provide for work intended to build health.

The World Health Organisation's (WHO) 'classic' statement that:

> Health is a state of complete physical, mental and social well-being, and not merely the absence of disease or infirmity[3]

is still quoted in the health promotion literature as inspirational, despite setting its standards in such a way as to require health promoters to judge progress in their work against an unachievable absolute, and despite offering little to guide the resolution of questions about the actual and comparative values of the huge array of possible activities the generality of its formulation allows.

By contrast Seedhouse's ability-focused theory that:

> A person's optimum state of health is equivalent to the state of the set of conditions which fulfil or enable a person to work to fulfil his or her realistic chosen and biological potentials. Some of these conditions are of the highest importance for all people. Others are variable dependent upon individual abilities and circumstances . . .[4]

and his setting out of the nature of these central and other conditions, allows those who use this construction to develop a clear (albeit contentious, as all are) view of what constitutes health for individuals. This more practicable formulation allows the making of justifiable decisions about health-promoting activities.

This example notwithstanding, many health promotion writings either directly or indirectly indicate health as the goal of health promotion, and although some proceed from a discussion of the meaning of health to attempts to elucidate a rationale for health promotion, a common feature of these accounts is that the meaning they give to 'health' is too vague to provide an adequate basis for evaluating the actions of health promoters. It is sometimes even advanced that the meaning of health promotion is uncertain or elusive and that disputes over meaning should not be permitted to hinder its pursuit.[5] Often it seems that 'the meaning of health' is allowed a touchstone quality which enables all to agree that health is something valuable and therefore to be pursued, without the need to concur on the essential nature of the value it provides, nor to tailor the practical pursuit accordingly.

'Well-being' as Purpose

Commonly, it is agreed that health is something more than the absence of disease and illness and that this 'more than' can be encapsulated in some notion of 'well-being'. Where accounts of 'health' are too vague, or are seen as too medical, 'well-being' is introduced as the essential quality upon which the purposive claims of health promotion are founded. But, given its basically practical nature, the health promotion 'movement' might be expected to be able to demonstrate more than a commitment to some kind of intuitive truth. At the very least we might expect that if 'well-being' is potentially an ambiguous term the possibilities for ambiguity will have been removed by commitment to and use of a particular meaning.

The source of much 'well-being speak' in health promotion theory is the WHO. Thus it is reasonable to look to the WHO for evidence of a unitary and clear account of 'well-being' as the purposive root for health promotion. The following statements are taken from one WHO paper:[6]

> Health and well-being are improved through the complex interactions of initiatives in various sectors.

> Public health is the science and art of promoting health. It does so based on the understanding that health is a process engaging social, mental, spiritual and physical well-being.

> As health—social, physical, mental and spiritual well-being—is the outcome of societal pattern, improved health in a society provides information on the general quality of life (context) and the *overall* values (meaning) of the society.

Without proceeding to pick through the bones of these statements, it is evident that the different constructions of the relationship between 'health' and 'well- being' they contain do *not* indicate the existence of a clear, unitary view. Overall the WHO literature offers scant evidence of a well-developed philosophically consistent account of 'well-being'. At best, its articulation is confused and poor.

Attempts to develop a sustainable 'well-being account', building from the WHO's jumbled and largely rhetorical usage, have been hampered by the traditional faith placed in synthesis as the path to clarity (that is, by the historical willingness of health promotion theorists to allow everyone into the temple). Downie, Fyfe and Tannahill's attempt is typical.[7] It founders on the assumption that health promotion must retain disease/illness (its historical base) as a privileged element in the account, while also arguing that health promotion is much more than medical work. These theorists thus enter a trap where they are forced to identify more than one purpose for health promotion—disease prevention (or, as they say, the prevention of 'negative health'), and the creation of 'true well-being' and 'fitness' (which they call 'positive health'). They conclude that there is a 'lack of a clear predictable relationship between negative and positive health' whilst also acknowledging that ultimately a coherent purposive account of health promotion can only be achieved by the reconciliation of the two 'based on value judgements'.

In effect their account concedes the frailty of its own construction through its inability to identify meaningfully the metric for this reconciliation, i.e. to be able to say clearly what the ultimate purpose of health promotion *is*, and so to be able to arbitrate in cases where purposes conflict.

Towards a Philosophical Basis for Health Promotion

Health promotion has failed to set out a view of 'well-being' which goes much beyond the intuitive. It certainly has not identified a unified theoretical base to allow it to assess its activities. The question remains whether such an account is possible.

Given that philosophers have developed a variety of accounts of 'well-being', some 'subjective' and others 'objective', it should perhaps be no surprise that a uniform view has not emerged. But this situation is quite unsatisfactory given the implicit claims of health promotion to be an unambiguous movement.

What form would an account need to take to allow a practical relationship between process and purpose to emerge? To begin with, any account which ultimately places health promotion purpose in a hedonistic conception can be dismissed as a poor option. Although such accounts might have appeal since they appear to give a single quality to assess (happiness, say) the appeal is superficial. Those dimensions to subjective well-being assessments which are to do with the exercise of individual reason and choice (i.e. those very qualities commonly seen as required for individuals to conceive of a good life for themselves) inhibit the possibility of a consistently practical relationship emerging between provision and *achieved* subjective well-being as happiness, simply because different people achieve happiness in different ways. This problem, of a claim extended beyond the chain of what is practically possible, applies also to the option of using simple preference satisfaction as a proxy for well-being. To do so would make health promotion's claims unbounded and any attempts to compare the validity of different possible activities an exercise in futility.

Unreserved acceptance of subjective accounts of 'well-being' as purpose would, for example, mean that if my experience of alcohol consumption is that drinking beyond the 'recommended limits' makes me happy (or that my sense of 'well-being' would be enhanced by measures which would make the exercise of my preference easier, say a reduction in alcohol duty levels or a relaxation in the licensing hours), then support to enable me to achieve higher consumption would count as health promotion work. So too would work towards increasing alcohol duty and more stringent licensing laws in response to the contradictory subjective experiences of others. In such a case health promotion would be without direction.

The absurdity of any 'movement' holding this sort of position is reflected in the fact that health promotion does *not* unreservedly welcome subjective accounts of 'well-being' as defining its goal, but moves to judge some of these accounts as incomplete or deviant, and so to exclude them. Only the happiness generated by conservative drinking behaviour is recognised as genuine and only those activities intended to stimulate low consumption are seen to count as health promotion.

This filtering means that, despite the popular expression of its purpose in such terms, health promotion accords little status to individual judgements of 'well-being'. Even for those activities the movement currently accepts as health promoting, few efforts are made to show the existence of causal relationships between their introduction and the consistent creation of felt 'well-being' in the individuals or groups targeted, which the persistence of claims to a practical and clear relationship should demand.

Objective Health Promotion?

Talk of filters or of limits to the acceptance of subjective accounts of 'well-being' is in effect to speak of an essentially objective (or external, or prejudiced) account of 'well-being', which will inevitably involve an element of 'moral imperialism'. If subjective accounts are to be rejected as a viable option for health promotion's account of purpose on the grounds of impracticality, what form would this alternative objective account need to display? It too would need to avoid the impracticality trap, so it would need to offer some sustainable support to the claim that health promotion's activities can actually achieve the specified form of 'well-being'. At the same time it would have to retain as a key defining feature the freedom of individuals to make choices as to how to pursue their own lives and judge their experiences (to do otherwise would be to accept that individuals' feelings about their own lives generally offer less reliable accounts than the imagined interpretations of second parties). In effect, an 'objective account' would need to prescribe those *means* it says to be enabling and protective of this capacity to make choices, and would have to be able to explain all health promotion activities in such terms. It would have to assert that:

1. Access to a set of means identified as commonly required to satisfy an appropriate minimum level and range of choice opportunity for all people should be provided.
2. Access to choice opportunity for each individual beyond (1), to reflect the specific choices made by individuals as a function of (1), should be provided.

The claim to a unitary account should be sustained through such a descripton of purpose, and the possibility of demonstrating the relationship between this purpose and health promotion's process activities (and for comparative and aggregative measurement) would be allowed by the existence of a single quality—'capacity for self-direction'. Although the value attached to diverse activities would clearly be the subject of a process of vigorous debate, the focus of the debate would be clear and the question 'what activities should qualify as health promotion?' defined by that focus rather than obscured by custom, habit or prejudice.

A rich literature of philosophical accounts of 'health', 'well-being', 'welfare' and 'quality of life'[8–10] is emerging which could assist the process of building a more specific purposive account for health promotion. Unless this opportunity is taken health promotion will continue to lose sight of health in the contingent concerns of provision.

References

1. Noack, H. (1985). Concepts of health and health promotion. In, *Measurement in Health Promotion and Protection*, WHO, Regional Office for Europe and International Epidemiological Association.
2. Nutbeam, D. (1985). *Health Planning Glossary*, WHO, Regional Office for Europe.
3. World Health Organisation. (1946). *Constitution*, WHO, Geneva.
4. Seedhouse, D.F. (1986). *Health: The Foundations for Achievement*, John Wiley & Sons, Chichester.
5. Ashton, J. and Seymour, H. (1988). *The New Public Health*, Open University Press, Milton Keynes.
6. Kickbush, I. (1989). *Good Planets are Hard to Find*, WHO, Regional Office for Europe.
7. Downie, R.S., Fyfe, C. and Tannahill, A. (1990). *Health Promotion Models and Values*, Oxford University Press, Oxford.
8. Nordenfelt, L. (1987). *On the Nature of Health. An Action–Theoretic Approach*, D. Reidel, Dordrecht.
9. Sen, A. (1982). *Choice, Welfare and Measurement*, Basil Blackwell, Oxford.
10. Griffin, J. (1986). *Well-being*, Oxford University Press, Oxford.

Conclusion

Theory before Practice?

This book has described a range of practical health reform projects, and has (in the introduction) made it clear that to make sense of these projects, and to see why they do not and cannot fully work, it is necessary to comprehend the underlying logic of reform. However it is also apparent that logic alone is not enough to guide meaningful, coherent health reform. A developed and justified theory of health is required too.

It is further evident that although theories of health can be derived in part from purely conceptual analysis, any theory of health must be connected in some way with a broader social or political philosophy. The contributions to Part Two illustrate this point very well. Stuart Spicker's proposal for practical health reform is replete with references to social philosophy, as is Michael Loughlin's response. If anything Erich Loewy makes the importance of social philosophy more obvious still as he calls for a fundamental shift in American social planning—demanding a move from individualism to a greater emphasis on community, and arguing that only if the American social ethos changes can practical health reform radically address people's needs. The Dutch, of course, already have a 'communitarian philosophy' but—as is the case with any social philosophy—this too has its detractors.

Quite clearly the health reform debate must take place at two overlapping levels. There are questions of pragmatics: how can we save money? How can we make sure that everyone at least gets some help? How can we regulate the role of commerce in health care? How can we give choice to health professionals and to patients? And there are questions of social philosophy: should the health system reflect libertarian or communitarian values? Should the state plan the health system equitably or should the system be 'designed' by the market? Where health services have to be rationed should they be allocated on the basis of need or should they be provided first where they can be most cost-effective? Both sets of questions must be addressed in any intelligent discussion of health reform, but often only one or other set (usually the set of practical issues) is considered. But both aspects are essential, and can be united by means of well-formulated theories of health.

Reforming Health Care: The Philosophy and Practice of International Health Reform.
Edited by D. Seedhouse. © 1995 John Wiley & Sons Ltd.

Starting with Theory rather than Practice

It is quite apparent that there are enormous conceptual and practical problems associated with international health reform, and that one of the main sources of these difficulties is the lack of a proper theory of health. Since the purpose of health systems is universally supposed to be the creation of health, since the nature of health is obscure, and since the *purpose* of health systems and the *systems themselves* are dependent variables, the present function of the various systems acts to define the system's goals. And since the system itself is internally inconsistent (as witnessed by all contributors to Part One) so too is the 'theory' it generates.

The main benefit (if it is right to call this a benefit) of having the system 'define' the theory rather than the other way round is that the size of the system is contained. That is, since what *is* entirely defines what *ought to be*, the system has been allowed to build its own boundary. Furthermore, since one of the main reasons—and in some places the only reason—for health reform is the restriction of financial cost it suits some governments perfectly to know that the health system is almost universally conceived of in a way that means that it limits itself.

However, this apparently welcome expedience has the implication that health reform as presently conceived cannot be a logical matter. Because much of what is believed to comprise 'health systems' is arbitrary and contingent (the emphasis on hospitals rather than community care, medicine's higher status in comparison to other forms of human support), and because there is no proper account of the purpose of health systems, then to try to restructure a health system along rational lines is bound to fail. Whatever suggestion for reform is made it will inevitably have detractors (those who 'lose out' in some way from the rearrangements are certain to protest), and however hard the reformers try to justify the rearrangement they will never be able to come up with finally convincing reasons to account for them because the question of health system purpose is so obscure at present—in other words, without philosophical underpinning, any reforms are bound to appear to be motivated by one political reason or another. Reforms will seem to be to do either with internal health service politics, with party politics, or with broader ideological concerns. And this, in every case to date, is undoubtedly what the 90s 'health reforms' have actually been.

How might things look if reforms were driven not by the system but by a worked through notion of health? The full discussion of theories and definitions of health is beyond the scope of this book, but it is possible to indicate how much hangs on it. The framework of a theory of health has been drawn by the case study in Part Three. Between them Nordenfelt, Cribb, Dougherty and Buchanan have described what is lacking from the philosophy of health promotion, and so have indicated the essential features that any theory of health must have. To make philosophical sense a theory of health must set clear limits (there must be borders beyond which it does not apply), it must say what the goals of health work are, and it must say how the processes of health work are compatible with, and can actually produce, health as defined by the theory.

Without a theory of health (and, as Dougherty argues, without a theory that can define the limits of people's responsibility) not only are we unable to tell what health promotion work is, but also we can have no way of knowing whether health promotion interventions have been successful (if we don't know what health is, how can we measure the results of work designed to promote it?).

There is, of course, much more to the philosophy of health promotion than can be demonstrated in this book. However, it should be clear enough that what applies in the case of health promotion must also apply in the case of health reform. Without a theory of health reform it is difficult if not impossible to understand health reform beyond the level of pragmatics (cost-control, professional rivalries, governments keen to shape social institutions according to favoured political views, and so on). And without a philosophical theory it is certainly impossible to measure the success of health reforms in a way removed from the more mundane political arguments.

Broad and Narrow Theories of Health

Consider two theories of health, the one broad, the other narrow. Assume that the narrow theory says that a person is healthy when she has no physical disease, when she is reasonably fit, when she is not injured, when she has no disability, and when she is not depressed or over-anxious. And assume that the broad theory claims that:

> A person's optimum state of health is equivalent to the state of the set of conditions which fulfil or enable a person to work to fulfil his or her realistic chosen and biological potentials. Some of these conditions are of the highest importance for all people. Others are variable dependent upon individual abilities and circumstances.[1]

> (Which means roughly that a reasonably healthy person will have a fairly extensive range of opportunities in life, will be able to develop creatively, and will not be suffering from a greatly disabling life obstacle.)

What would the implications for health reform be if one or the other of these theories were to be in the 'driving seat'? On both the narrow and the broad account of health, there would be a major effect on the 'health system' (see Figure 1). All the outer boxes in the figure have a part to play in ensuring the achievement of even the narrowest view of health. Clearly such aspects of life as jobs, pollution and road dangers have an effect on a person's health even if 'health' is defined to mean clinically recognisable problems only. The broader view acknowledges the logic of this, and simply requires that all the functions of a government concerned to promote the health of all its people should be designed in order to maximise citizens' chances of having fulfilling lives, free from as many impediments to their creative movement as possible.

Whatever the scope of a theory of health chosen to act as the philosophical *raison d'être* for health reform, its effect must be to break down the existing edifice.[2] At the moment health reforms are seen as 'those things that can be done

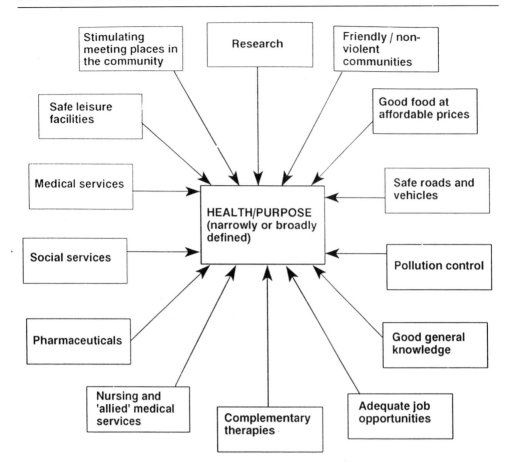

The Health System governed by a theory of health

Figure 1 Whether a 'broad' or 'narrow' theory of health is used to guide health reform a great deal more is drawn into the health system (boxes an illustrative sample only)

to improve the existing system' (and it has already been seen in the Introduction how this 'internal logic' collapses) whereas if reforms were to be driven by a theory of health, reform would of necessity be seen as 'those things that can be done to improve the nation's health'. Of course, this change of emphasis removes none of the controversy about the nature of health, and nor does it make it any easier to assess the outcomes of 'health interventions'. Indeed, if work for health is thought to be work to ensure as much fulfilling life for everyone then its precise measurement is almost certainly impossible.

On the other hand, if reforms were to begin with theory rather than assume that the structures that actually exist are the best attainable, rational planning would at least be a possibility. Medical systems would not be protected by the assumption that 'most nations spend around 7–8% of their wealth on medical services therefore so should we', but their costs and benefits would have to be assessed alongside those of other measures that nations might take to improve the health of their citizens. At the very least, the reform of 'the health system' according to this notion of purpose would require that the traditionally defined 'health system' (medical services) would have to compete for resources with those services and processes that are not currently defined as part of the health system, but which would enter the health system given this notion of purpose. And, on a rational system, the medical system would succeed in gaining resources to the extent to which it could contribute to the broad notion of health (so far as this could be measured).

All this is beginning to sound very much like a message from the philosophical map-maker—logical, but idealistic and so unobtainable. But what is the alternative? There is, at the moment, an international conviction that it is time to improve health systems. There have already been many attempts to do this, and each has run into trouble. Analysis shows that these problems were entirely predictable (for the reasons given in the Introduction and this concluding chapter) and that unless reforms begin from theory rather than convention they cannot succeed (if for no other reason because, as things stand, the nature of success is bound to be disputed).

Of course it is obvious that *some* reforms to 'health systems' are possible. If a sub-system is defined as 'the use of technology' then reform to this system across those hospitals where the reformer has authority could cut out surplus machines and redirect resources (although this redirection would have to be done according to a broader notion of purpose). Clearly, where there is obvious waste something can be done about it (and especially if 'cost-control' is actually the dominant purpose). But, equally clearly, it is one thing to prevent the blatant squandering of resources that might be used elsewhere, and quite another to reform all sub-systems, logically, according to a clearly defined overall purpose.

Without doubt health reform is highly desirable. And there will probably never be a better time to achieve it than now. However, health reforms cannot work unless the reformers understand the logic and philosophy of health reform. If health reform is seriously intended health reformers have no choice but to get the overall theory in place as soon as possible.

References

1. Seedhouse, D.F. (1986). *Health: The Foundations for Achievement*, John Wiley & Sons, Chichester.
2. Seedhouse, D.F. (1994). *Fortress NHS: A Philosophical Review of the National Health Service*, John Wiley & Sons, Chichester.

Index

Acquired immune deficiency syndrome
  (AIDS) 114
Age-related conditions 23
Ageing population 23–4
Agency for Healthcare Policy and
  Research 17
Aid to Families with Dependent
  Children (AFDC) 27, 46–7
Altman, Lawrence K. 131
American Disabilities Act (ADA) 39
American Farm Bureau Federation 61
American Medical Association (AMA)
  60
ANC national health plan 112–16
Apartheid 101–7
Audit Commission 75
Australia 62
Autonomy 158, 169–70, 193, 195, 204

Baby boom generation 23
Balance-billing 67
Bantu Affairs Administration Boards
  106
Bantu peoples 108
Bartlett, Will 79
Beneficence 158
Bimodal health care 152–3
Birch, Bill 89
Blue Cross/Blue Shield plan 66
Boston, J. 88
Bristol and Weston Health Authority
  79
British Medical Association 177
Budgeting systems
  global budget 62
  The Netherlands 161
  United States 25
Butler, John 74

Califano, Joseph 60
Callahan, Daniel 50, 51, 163
Canada 21, 22, 60–9

financing national health care 67–9
history of public health insurance 60
national health insurance, basic outline
  63–4
quality of health care 65
rationing care 64–5
Canadian National Health Insurance:
  Lessons for the United States 60
Capron, Alexander 44, 49, 50
Care
  culture of 174, 178
  nature of 177–80
Charity care 131–2
Charter of Patients' Rights 115
Children, health promotion in 194
Cigarette smoking
  and socio-economic status 215
  during pregnancy 215
Citizens' Health Care Parliament 29
Clarke, Kenneth 74, 77, 78
Clinton, President Bill 62
  see also Clinton health reform plan
Clinton health reform plan 53–9
  administrative simplification 59
  basic challenge to 55
  fallback position 54
  federal framework options 59
  financial security vs ideal system
    57–9
  reshaping the administrative design
    59
  theoretical difficulties 54–5
  workability 55–7
Clinton, Hillary Rodham 54
Commercial systems
  reforming 3–4
  basic contours of 4
Commodification 177
Community, alternative vision 157–9
Community Health Centres 104–5
Community-oriented approach 98–9,
  162–3

Community rating 20
Community values 31–3
Competition 62, 138, 150, 156, 176, 177
Conflicting issues 5, 8
Continental Divide 61
Coronary bypass surgery 156
Costs
    health care 15–16, 149, 161
    The Netherlands 161
    United States 15–16
Criminality in health promotion 195
Crown Health Enterprises (CHEs) 87,
    89, 90

Dalziel, P. 88
Daniels, N. 98, 156
Danzon, P. 88, 89
Davis, James E. 131
de Beer, C. 105, 106, 108
Dementia 23
Dental services 32
Department of Health and Human
    Services (DHHS) 49–51, 58
Diagnostic Related Groups (DRGs) 48
District health authorities 81
Dobson, Frank 73
Downie, R.S. 224
Drug addiction 196

Eastern Europe 167
Efficiency 174–5, 177
Elderly persons 23–4
Employment-based health insurance 24,
    135
Engelhardt, H.T. 154
Enterprise culture 178
Enthoven, A. 74, 137, 138
Environmental factors 213
Ethical issues 178
    alternative vision 157–9
    existential *a prioris* 158
    'haves' vs 'have nots' 131–4
    healthfare state 137–9
    in health promotion 189–96, 201
    moral critique 145–7
    New Zealand 90
    Oregon health care project 43–51
Evans, Bob 60
Existential *a prioris* of ethics 158

Facticity Model 210

and victim-blaming 213–14
vs freedom model 216–18
Family Health Service Authority 75
Fourie, A. 107
France, health insurance 62
Free health care 131
Free market system 167, 170
Freedom Model 210
    and health promotion 211–13
    vs facticity model 216–18
Fudging 5
Fund-holding general practitioners 72,
    79–82
Fyfe, C. 224

Garrison, William L. 117
General practitioners, fund-holding 72,
    79–82
Genetic factors 213, 214
Germany
    and former East Germany 167–70
    consequences of 'overnight' break with
        traditions and habits 169–70
    decentralised system 21
    governmental role 62
    health care reform 169
    health insurance 62
Gibbs, Alan 88, 89
Ginzberg, E. 133
Glennerster, H. 79
Global budget 62
Gluckman Commission 104
Gluckman, H. 104, 105
Golenski, John 29, 45
Goodin, R.E. 133
Gore, Senator Albert Jr. 39
Green and White Paper 86, 87
Griffiths Report 74
Gross domestic product (GDP) 15
Gross national product (GNP) 62, 132,
    150
Group Areas Act 1950 103
Guide to the Health Act 1978 109
Guillebaud Committee 73

Hadorn, D.C. 46
Hawaii 20
Health
    classic statement 223
    concept of 197
    determinants of 207

individual responsibility for   211
'middle range' conception   203
notion of   186, 187, 230
theories of   10–11, 229–33
welfare conception of   206
Health Act   1977 105, 108
Health Alliances   57
Health care
    costs   15–16, 149, 161
    criteria for setting priorities   164–5
    expenditure   161
    South Africa   107
    necessary   162–3
    needs   97–8, 134–6
    non-essential   162
    rationing. *See* Rationing health care
    relationships   179, 180
Health care reform
    characterisation of   7
    conceptual and practical problems
        associated with   230
    contemporary view   7
    evaluation   171–82
    extrinsic and intrinsic evaluation
        172–5
    logic of   1–2
    'macro' and 'micro' perspectives   174
    nature of   2–11
    philosophy and practice   1–2
    process and outcome   7
    prospects for   11
    theory-based   10
Health education   192
Health insurance   17–18, 20, 29, 131,
    134–6, 162
    and employment   135
Health Insurance Association of America
    (HIAA)   60, 61
Health Maintenance Organisations
    (HMO)   54, 131
Health of the Nation   80
Health promotion   185–97
    action-theoretical context   201
    and disease management   204
    and disease prevention   206–7
    and Freedom Model   211–13
    and goal of health   186–7
    and individual control   214–16
    and normal basic drives   196
    borders of   203–7
    collective actions   185–6
    compulsion   193–7
    criminality in   195
    deliberate   202
    direct   186, 187, 189–90
    ethical issues   189–96, 201
    forms of   187–9
    framing interventions   205–6
    general utility argument   189
    implicit claims of   222
    in children   194
    in mentally handicapped persons   194
    in senile persons   194
    indirect   186–8, 190–2
    individual actions   185
    institutional actions   185–6
    intention condition   200–3
    interactive   201
    limits of   209–20
    meaning of   199–200
    objective   226
    pattern of development   221
    philosophy of   200, 225–6, 231
    policy framework   218–19
    prohibition   193
    public policy   204–5
    purposes and processes   222–3
    societal or institutional measures   192
    South Africa   115
    specific categories   189–92
    use of term   199
    well-being of   223–6
    WHO advocacy   207
    WHO literature   204, 224
Health protection   192
Health status and individual behaviour
    209
Health system   230
    interpretation of   8
    overall desired purposes   8
    sub-system purposes   8
    super-purpose   10
Healthfare state
    ethical critique   137–9
    moral dilemma   136
    prudential and ethical critique   131–41
Healthy People   211
Healthy People 2000   211
Heart surgery   124
Heart transplantation   110
    South Africa   110
Heroic medicine   18

Hip fractures   23
Hobbes, Thomas   153, 154
Home health care   25
Homelessness   147, 170
Human immunodeficiency virus (HIV)
    114

Iacocca, Lee   60
Individual approach   164
Individual behaviour and health status
    209
Individual consumer perspective   164
Individual control and health promotion
    214–16
Individual freedom   138, 139
    vs social intelligence   139
Individual responsibility for health   211
Information systems, South Africa   111
Information technology   74
Informed consent   191
Inquiry into the Nature and Causes of the
    Wealth of Nations, An   133
Institute of Family and Community
    Medicine   105
Internal Revenue Service (IRS)   138
in vitro fertilisation (IVF)   162
Ischaemic heart disease   156

Japan   62

Kennedy, Senator Ted   60
Kerry, Senator   61
King's Fund Institute   177
Kitzhaber, Senator John   29, 45
Knowles, John   211
Kronick, R.   137, 138

Land Act   1913 103
Legislation   192, 193
    South Africa   103
Le Grand, Julian   79, 80, 133
Libertarianism   154
Lifecare corporation   109
Life-style risk factors   211–12
Lippmann, Walter   139
Lipset, Seymour Martin   61
Lithuania   121–7
    asymmetry between specialised and
        primary health care   124
    economic crisis   123
    medical equipment   124

medical personnel   124
National Conception of Health   125–6
present situation   124–5
preventive medicine   126
primary health care institutions   124
private clinics and pharmacies   124
rationing criteria   125
reorganising health care   125
resource allocation   121–3
self-imposed conceptual challenge
    125–6
tipping rates   124–5
transition of health care   121
Long-term care   24, 25
Loram Commission   103

Macara, A.W.   177
MacIntyre, A.   179
Macleod, Iain   73
Magaziner, Ira   54
Magnetic resonance imaging (MRI)   25,
    155–6
Major, John   76
Malpractice insurance coverage   16, 131
Mammogram machines   16
Managed competition   62, 138
Market economy in health care   74
Market forces   74–5, 150, 154–5
Maynard, A.   176
McKinseys   73
Medicaid
    beneficiaries   29
    comparison with Medicare   27–8
    expenditure   47, 49
    extended access   18, 20, 22–3, 30, 68,
        136
    funding   29, 37, 44
    government outlays   15, 19, 21, 23
    integration with Medicare   44
    limited access   17, 18, 27, 45, 102
    nursing home coverage   24
Medical Association of South Africa
    105
Medical audit   82
Medical education   16
Medical professional approach   164
Medicare
    Canadian experience   60–2
    comparison with Medicaid   27–8
    elderly persons' coverage   47, 58
    extended access   23

funding 29
  government outlays 15, 21, 132
  integration with Medicaid 44
Medico-biological perspective 164
Mental health and chemical dependency
  (MHCD) 31, 32, 48
Mentally handicapped persons, health
  promotion 194
Menzel, Paul 49, 50
Monheit, Alan C. 135
Moore, John 72, 74
Moral critique 145–7
Moral reasoning 143
Mortality rates, South Africa 106–7
Motivation of health care professionals
  178

National Advisory Committee on Core
  Health and Disability Support
  Services (NACCHDS) 87
National Association of Health
  Authorities 78
National Centre for Health Services
  Research and Health Care
  Technology
  Assessment (NCHSR) 135
National Commission of Health
  Technology 115
National Health Board (NHB) 57, 58
National Health Service (NHS) 71
  background influences 72–4
  commercial competition 177
  competition in 74–5, 176
  confidential review team 73–4
  consumer voice in post-reform 82
  evaluating health market reforms
    175–7
  evaluation of reforms 79–80
  fund-holding general practitioners 72,
    79–82
  hospital trusts 77
  income generation schemes 73
  internal market 77–9, 171, 176, 177
  local plans 77
  Management Executive 78
  market forces 74–5
  medical opposition 78
  opposition to government's proposals
    76
  over-bureaucratisation of reforms 81
  priorities 80–1

  proposals and legislation 74–7
  tension between market freedom and
    government regulation 81
  tension between medical professionals,
    managers and consumers 81
  tensions resulting from reforms 80–3
  traditional values vs. business values
    180
  'trust' hospitals 72
National railway system, reform process
  4–6
Ncayiyana, D.J. 112
NEHAWU 109
Netherlands, The 88, 91, 95–100
  access to services 99
  balance between individual interests
    and general welfare 96
  basic health care needs 97–8
  Committee on Choices in Health Care
    162, 163
  community-oriented approach to
    health 98–9
  criteria for setting priorities 162, 163
  fundamental approach to core health
    services 96–7
  health care costs 161
  health care resource allocation 95
  individual approach to health 98
  insurance programme 162
  medical professional approach to
    health 98
  options to reduce pressure on health
    care system 96–7
  principle of solidarity 99
  public debate on health care services
    99
  strategies for making health care
    choices 98–9
New Zealand
  competitive market model 88
  core health services 91
  ethical issues 90
  funding of primary care services 86
  health expenditure 86
  health system prior to reforms 86
  implications of health care reforms
    89–92
  main features of health care reforms
    87
  purchaser/provider split 92
  quality of service 91

New Zealand (*cont.*)
  restructuring of health services 85–94
  theoretical and ideological
    underpinnings 87–8
Newton, Tony 73
NHS. *See* National Health Service
  (NHS)
NHS and Community Care Act 1990
  71, 78, 175
NHS Trust Federation 81
Nordenfelt, Lennart 200, 201, 202, 203,
  204, 206
Normal functioning 162–3, 164
Nozick, R. 154
Nursing homes 24

OBHSA. *See* Oregon Basic Health
  Services Act 1989 (OBHSA)
On the Nature of Health 186
Oregon Basic Health Benefits Act 30
Oregon Basic Health Services Act 1989
  (OBHSA) 30–44
Oregon Health Action Council 32
Oregon health care project 22–3, 27–52
  background 27–9
  chronology of key events in
    prioritisation 28
  community values 31–3
  ethical issues 43–51
  final approval 43
  health outcomes assessment 33–4
  opposing arguments 46
  prioritisation lists 34–43
  prioritisation plan 44
  responses to DHHS 49–51
Oregon Health Council 29
Oregon Health Decisions Inc. (OHD)
  29
Oregon Health Insurance Partnership
  Act 30
Oregon Health Services Commission
  (HSC) 29
  subcommittees and models 31
Oregon Medicaid Priority-Setting
  Project (MPP) 29, 31
Oregon State Health Risk Pool 30
Organ transplantation 124
Organisation for European Co-operation
  and Development 62

Pan Africanist Congress (PAC) health

  policy 116–17
Paternalism 191, 193, 197
Patient education 16
Patient's Charter 76, 80
Physician Payment Review Commission
  (PPRC) 58
Physicians for a National Health Plan
  (PNHP) 61
'Play or pay' system 20
Positron emission tomography (PET)
  156
Poverty
  and negative attitudes 215–16
  statistics 150–3
  vs being poor 151–2
Practical syllogism 188, 190, 192,
  195
Preferred provider organisations (PPO)
  131
Pregnancy, cigarette smoking during
  215
Preventive medicine
  and health promotion 205
  ethical issues 187
  Germany 169–70
  Lithuania 126
  Oregon 32, 48
  United States 16
Prioritisation of Health Services 31
Private health care 181
Private health insurance 21
Private patients 90
Private practice, South Africa 109–10
Private sector, South Africa 109
Professional autonomy 181
Profit maximisation 3–5
Prospective Payment Commission for
  hospitals (PROPAC) 58
Protestantism 153
Prudential critique 131–41, 143–5
Prudential reasoning 143
Public Health Commission 87
Public Service Labour Relations Act
  1993 109

Quality Adjusted Life Years (QALYs)
  46, 48
Quality assurance 56
Quality of life 226
Quality of Well-Being Scale (QWB) 31,
  33, 34, 39, 48, 50

Ranade, Wendy 77
Rationing health care 174, 175
  Canada 64–5
  Lithuania 125
Reform
  basic contours of 6
  conditions for 2–3
  definition 2, 5
  practical conditions for 11
  questions to the reformer 3
  see also Health care reform
Regional health authorities (RHAs) 76,
  78, 87, 89–92
Resource allocation 161
  Lithuania 121–3
  The Netherlands 95
Resource Management Institute (RMI)
  74
Responsibility for nation's health
  167–70
  former East Germany 169
  possible bases 167–8
  socialist understanding of 168–9
Restructuring, of sub-systems 3–4
Risk adjustment 56
Risk rating 20
Rousseau, J.J. 157

Schopenhauer, A. 157
Schur, Claudia L. 135
Seedhouse, D.F. 223
Senile persons, health promotion 194
Shalala, Donna 43
Sheps, Cecil 60
Sickness funds 21
Single-payer system 24, 25
Sipes-Metzler, Paige 43
Skocpol, Theda 57
Slabber, C.F. 107
Smith, Adam 133–4, 144, 145, 153, 157
Social deprivation and ill-health 144
Social intelligence 139
  vs individual freedom 139
Social policies 133
Social relations 173–5
Socialised medicine 19
Society Must Decide 29
Socio-economic status and cigarette
  smoking 215
South Africa 101–19
  advisory bodies 108

ANC national health plan 112–16
apartheid 101–7
basic level health care 108
constraints on health policy planning
  110–11
damage to health care services 109
drug policy 115
early historical distortion of health and
  health care 102–3
health promotion 115
heart transplantation 110
hospital bed occupancy rates 107
inequality in provision of health
  services 106–7
information systems 111
lack of coordination of health care
  108
legislation 103
mental health 115–16
misleading propaganda 108
mortality rates 106–7
National Health Services Commission,
  1942–1944 104–5
Nationalist regimes 103
Pan Africanist Congress (PAC) health
  policy 116–17
per capita expenditure on health 107
population growth 111
private practice 109–10
private sector 109
process and nature of change 111–12
racist distortions of health and health
  care 103
traditional healers 116
unconscious racism 103
South African Medical Journal 110,
  112
Spicker, S.F. 143–7
Subsidiation 136, 138
Sub-systems 8
  reforming 3
  restructuring 3–4
Sullivan, Louis 39
Suppression of Communism Act 1950
  103

Tannahill, A. 224
Taskforce on Hospitals and Related
  Services 88
Tax credits 136
Taxation 24

Technology 149, 150, 155–7
Thatcher, Margaret 71, 72, 74
Towards a Theory of Health Promotion
    186
Traditional culture 175
Traditional healers, South Africa 116
Traditional health care ethics 174
Troughton, Peter 89
Tuberculosis 102, 109

Unemployment insurance 20, 22, 135,
    151, 170
Unemployment statistics 151
United Kingdom (UK) 62, 71–84
    restructuring of Welfare State 71
    see also National Health Service
    (NHS)
United States health care
    adapting Canada's health care system
        66–7
    and Canadian experience 60–9
    and Canadian model 69
    and social conditions 150
    comprehensive reform 19
    conditions 150–3
    employment-based insurance 24
    expenditure 15–16
    health insurance 17–18
    incremental revision 18–19
    limited access to 17–18
    mandated employer coverage 19–21
    national health insurance 21–2, 24
    planning for the future 23–4

prioritising services 23
proposed solutions 18–23
reform 15–26
reform debate 8–9
rising costs 15–16
setting priorities 22–3
see also Clinton health reform plan;
    Oregon health care project
Urban Areas Act 1923 103
USSR, former health care system
    121–3
Utilisation response 22

van Rensburg, H.C.J. 107
Victim-blaming 216–18, 218
von Wright, G.H. 188
Vorster, B.J. 105

Waxman, Senator Henry 39
Welfare conception 204
Welfare promotion 206
Welfare state 132–3
    'empirically' and 'conceptually' flawed
        143
Welfare systems 133
Well-being of health promotion 223–6
Wellington Health Action Committee
    88
Wilson, Harold 73
Wolfe, Sam 60
Working for Patients (White Paper) 72,
    74–6, 81, 82
Workplace coverage 20

Index compiled by Geoffrey C. Jones